DIET WITH VITAMINS

*The scientific guide to nutritionally
responsible weight-loss*

by DAVID P. RUBINCAM Ph.D.
and JOHN RUBINCAM

A & W PUBLISHERS, INC.
NEW YORK

This new and important book offers a fascinating concept for nutritional dieting. While the authors point out very clearly that their theory has not yet been
tested on vast numbers of people, the medical literature now available, they
believe, strongly supports their concepts.

If, however, one is under treatment for some ailment, it is best to consult
one's physician before entering upon this diet plan.

Published by
A & W Publishers, Inc.
95 Madison Avenue
New York, New York 10016.

Library of Congress Catalog Card Number: 77-73140
Designed by Bernard Schleifer
ISBN 0-89479-007-2

Printed in the United States of America

To Mom and Dad, and Milt III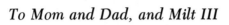

CONTENTS

1. An Introduction and Preview   1

Part I. The Nutrients

2. Vitamins and Minerals: The Forgotten
   Ingredients   9
3. Vitamin A: The Visible Vitamin   22
4. Vitamin C: Supervitamin?   29
5. Iron: Deficiency of Slow Suffocation   41
6. Calcium: Deficiency of Crumbling Bones   48
7. Thiamin: The First Vitamin   53
8. Niacin: Plucked from Confusion   58
9. Riboflavin: The Luminous Vitamin   62
10. Vitamin E: The Vitamin Protector   65
11. The Remaining Regulators: Iodine,
    Vitamin D, and Others   69
12. The Energy Nutrients and Fiber: Carbohydrates,
    Fat, Protein, and Cellulose   78

Part II: Energy and Overweight

13. On Becoming Fat: A Heritage from the Centuries   89
14. On Becoming Thin: Magic and Science   99

Part III: Reducing

15. How to Diet: Plan Number One   111
16. How to Diet: Plan Number Two   140
17. Exercise and Weight Reduction   155

Appendix: Nutritive Value of Foods   163
For Further Reading   257
A Note from the Author   259
Index   261

1

AN INTRODUCTION AND
PREVIEW

THE RIGHT WAY

Why do you want to lose weight?

If you're like most people, you want to reduce for two reasons, to improve your physical appearance, and to escape the medical liabilities associated with obesity.

And to do this, you'll turn either to a form of dieting, as the majority of persons interested in weight reduction do, or to some sort of exercise program, a possibility that attracts a smaller number of people.

But do you know how to diet, or what a good diet should contain, or what type of exercise to engage in to enable you to reach your goal?

Certainly there are many methods, many opinions from which to choose.

In fact, over the last thirty years the proliferation of diet and exercise schemes and ideas aimed at weight reduction has been incredible. One after another, year after year, they follow each other—and they all claim to be the last word in reducing! How so? If these boasts are true, why then are so many different procedures promoted?

The answer is simple—they don't work.

They fail to meet the needs of the reducer. Either they don't take off weight, or, if they do, they do it in a fashion that detracts from physical appearance and replaces the problems of overweight with disorders equally bad. Or at worst, they institute a combination of both, producing no weight loss as they damage looks and impair health.

Why don't they succeed?

Because they're based on nonsense, not science.

And as a scientist I'm amused at the bases for some of these diet plans and exercise programs, and appalled at the harm these systems can do. Their perpetrators do not understand how the human body operates. They don't know their science.

Why science to be successful in reducing?

Let me put it to you this way: If suddenly you had to go to Mars, would you depend on an astrologer to plot your route? Would you rely on the old diagrams and theories of Ptolemy, who thought the planets revolved around the earth? Or would you ask a present-day astronomer using computers to chart your course through the heavens? What if a loved one were deathly ill in Montreal, and you had to get there as fast as possible? Would you ask a mystic like Edgar Cayce to send you there? Would you go by horse and buggy? Or would you take the next jetliner out? And once you were in Montreal and they told you your loved one was endangered by polio, would you seek the consultation of a fortune teller? Would you demand a barber and an old-fashioned bloodletting? Or would you search out the advice and work of Jonas Salk and Albert Sabin, the scientists who conquered this dreaded disease?

When the chips are down, you know which way you'd go.

The astronomer and his computer. The jetliner. Salk and Sabin.

You'd choose science.

And you should do no less when you reduce.

For the process of sensible weight reduction, whether it is through dieting or exercise, falls into the provinces of nutritional and medical science, and for it to work it must be grounded in the fundamentals of biology, chemistry, and physics. In your quest to lose weight, you should look to the top scientists in the field, regarding closely the results of their studies, and not be taken in by the nutritional mystics or the dieting "barbers" who in effect wield rusty razors over your veins, distorting your nutritional needs to the point where you can be hurt, for there are penalties to pay if you should choose wrongly, as we shall see in the chapters ahead. The patient, the dieter, could take sick, or die.

Why not instead depend on the very best and latest research that the world of science has to offer?

Remember, science has one great advantage over all other approaches—it really works!

And it can be applied to reducing.

Science will tell us how to reduce; and by employing science, you will lose weight, improve your personal appearance, and add gains to your health.

And that is the purpose of this book—to help you lose weight without gambling your looks and well-being.

In it I present the method of reducing I've developed from proven scientific principles and documented technical studies. Meticulously calculated for your benefit (partly with the aid of a modern digital computer), this procedure centers around a system of dieting that keys in on the vitamins, other nutrients, and energy contained in natural foods.

I call it *the natural vitamin way*.

VITAMINS, REDUCING, AND THE GRAVEYARD

But why the emphasis on vitamins? What do they have to do with reducing?

The answer is that no nutrient can safely be ignored when you diet, whether it is one of the energy-producing nutrients— carbohydrate, fat, protein—or one of the body regulators, vitamins and their nutritional cousins, minerals. A diet, whether for reducing or not, should supply all of them. So in this sense I use vitamins as a symbol for every nutrient.

But vitamins in particular are indispensable to your diet and health—in fact, your life literally depends on their presence.

So vitamin intake should always be watched, especially so when you go on a weight-reduction diet that restricts eating in some fashion. For in this situation the likelihood that you'll obtain vitamins in the proper quantities is diminished. And that's bad. If you don't receive them in the right amounts, you can be disastrously hurt—by either too little or too much nutrition. For example, did you know that if you take in too few vitamins you court fatigue, headaches, nausea, anemia, insanity, and even death? Perhaps you were aware these things could happen. But did you also know that if you take vitamin pills as "insurance" you may still become a victim of deficiency? Or that if you ingest overly large numbers of pills you may lose your hair, damage your bones, or, if pregnant, risk giving birth to a mentally retarded child, or chance your own demise?

The possibilities are real. (I expound on them in the chapters to come.)

These problems have been well documented by medicine and nutritional science. Many persons have suffered from them, and in at least one instance a person has died from a nutritionally defective reducing diet—the Zen Macrobiotic Plan.

So if you think that dieting without regard to vitamins is dangerous, you're right! You must be careful. As you diet you don't want to trade the woes of obesity for nutritional ills that can be even more harmful to health and appearance.

So adequate provision for vitamins should be a part of any diet plan, and this holds true for all the nutrients.

Yet, when most people embark on a weight-loss program by dieting, they concern themselves only with limiting food intake in some way, and neglect the necessity of complete nutrition—to the deterioration of looks and health.

It is here, too, that the popular diet plans fail.

Enthralled with calories and the energy nutrients, they slight vitamins and minerals and the non-energy functions of carbohydrates, fat, and protein, or give you advice about them that can actually be injurious to your health—like the advocacy of massive doses of vitamin pills, or the declaration that carbohydrates are not good for you.

They forget about science.

But in this book we do not.

We use science to build an effective reducing method.

In *Part I: The Nutrients* we see exactly what a weight-reduction diet should contain, what should be left out, and what happens if we don't do as modern research dictates. *Part II: Energy and Overweight* explores the causes of obesity, the connection of energy to the problem, and how the balance of energy can be used to influence it. Drawing on all the previous information, *Part III: Reducing* outlines a scientific system of dieting for weight reduction and tackles the subject of exercise and its relation to losing weight, from the scientific viewpoint.

HIGHLIGHTS

In Chapter Two you'll discover why vitamins and minerals, the forgotten ingredients, are the most important part of any diet—far more vital than calories or carbohydrates. You'll glimpse the strange roles they play in keeping us alive and healthy, and you'll find out how their functions are affected by a reducing regimen. The chapter opens with a true-life scientific detective story that will convince you of the value of vitamins and minerals in sensible weight reduction.

We look at them individually in the next several chapters, closely scrutinizing the nutrients that are the most troublesome to dieters while showing you how to forestall the health and appearance problems they might cause as you reduce. It's here we talk about how much of each nutrient is enough, why it's dangerous to ingest excessively large doses of these powerful chemicals, and the best way to get the right amounts—natural foods or pills. You'll also be interested in what science has to say about those fabulous claims for vitamin C and cold prevention, and for vitamin E, the so-called sex vitamin. Are the claims valid, or not? Will dieting cheat you of any benefit?

Chapter Twelve reveals that the energy nutrients—carbohydrates, fat, protein—have functions beyond the providing of energy to the body, vital ones that can be interfered with by a weight-reduction diet. Even fat makes its contribution to body operation and cannot be ignored.

Chapter Thirteen details the real but little-known explanation of how and why people become fat in the first place. The reasons are rather startling, and you'll be surprised at the true source of obesity. And if you're one of the overweight, you'll be happy to learn that you're not to blame for your condition.

Once you have an understanding of the causes of obesity, we're ready to investigate the ways that surplus poundage can be eliminated. Magic, carbohydrates, and calories are discussed in Chapter Fourteen. Are there miracle remedies for corpulence that do not involve dieting or exercise? Do calories really count, and are carbohydrates actually more fattening than other foods? Calories versus carbohydrates—Chapter Fourteen discloses the truth about this century-old argument.

With Chapters Fifteen, Sixteen, and Seventeen we reach the culmination of the book.

In the first two of these chapters you'll see how to lose weight on the most comprehensive, flexible, and nutritious diet system ever devised. Constructed in part with the assistance of a modern digital computer, and centered on a core concept of maximum nutrition and precisely measured food energy, this plan insures rapid weight loss at the safest practical rate, guarantees optimal nutritional health, and is sound, painless, and permanent. Easy to follow, you'll find that *the natural vitamin way* is the only way to reduce by dieting.

We clear up a final muddy area in the realm of weight reduction in Chapter Seventeen with a little straight talk about exercise, a subject as controversial and confusing as the topic of dieting. Does exercise help or hinder the person attempting to lose weight? You'll know the answer after you read this chapter.

We begin our inquiry with a few thoughts on eating, after which we chase a killer across two continents.

That's in Chapter Two.

PART ONE

The Nutrients

2

VITAMINS AND MINERALS: THE FORGOTTEN INGREDIENTS

SUPPING

Have you ever stopped to think about why we eat?

Many of us would say that we consume food in order to satisfy a physical urge. We feel hunger, an emptiness, and eating helps to assuage this feeling. Of course, this line of reasoning is correct as far as it goes. But what is behind the desire itself, the phenomenon that makes us want to put food into our stomachs?

The answer is that in a sense man is a machine. And as a machine he needs fuel to run on, like an automobile needs gasoline. Man's fuel comes from food. And so he puts it into his stomach as we pump gasoline into a car's gas tank. But like the automobile, man requires other things besides fuel to operate effectively. If we don't add oil to our cars and replace worn spark plugs, the cars don't run well. And the same is true of man. He requires certain materials for his body to function properly. However, while automobiles get their lubricants and parts from factories, man receives the substances that allow him to operate efficiently from food, along with his fuel.

Now, anything in food that provides fuel, contributes material for building and maintenance of the body, or helps to regulate any body process is called a *nutrient*.

And it is here that dieting comes in.

By altering food intake in some way, such as decreasing it or limiting it to a certain selection of foods, dieting can play havoc with the nutrients the body needs. Usually, we're concerned with the energy nutrients: we'd like to lessen them or change their effect in some way to keep extra weight off the body. So we experiment with amounts and types of food. But in fooling with them we can also be tampering with the other nutrients, the regulators—to the detriment of health.

Specifically, I'm speaking of vitamins and minerals.

Vitamins and minerals in many ways are the most valuable nutrients; and you cannot afford to neglect them when you diet.

To see why, we begin their story with the tale of a mysterious killer, a dread disease, and of the medical detective, a doctor, who tracked it relentlessly across a country and faced it in its lair.

THE UNKNOWN FACTOR

In eighteenth-century Spain, reports of a strange disease came to the notice of doctors. The peasants afflicted with the disorder called it *mal de la rosa*—the red sickness—because they suffered painful, itching rashes on the parts of their skin exposed to the sun, mostly on the face and the hands. Also, their tongues became sore and red, and they frequently had an unslakable thirst. Headaches, abdominal pains, diarrhea, dizziness, and weakness were other complaints.

But *mal de la rosa* was not a disease of physical symptoms alone.

In addition, its victims suffered from mental disturbances. At the outset of the malady, the afflicted grew depressed and irritable; and, as time passed, they often fell into deep melancholy and had delusions of persecution and grievous sin. In the latter stages of the disease the victims deteriorated into unqualified madness. Death was commonly the final outcome.

The sickness spread through Europe, becoming prevalent in France and Italy where hospitals and asylums filled with its wretched prey. One insane asylum in Milan, housing five hundred lunatics, could boast that two-thirds were there because the red malady had driven them mad.

Frapoli, an Italian physician studying the disease, renamed it *pellagra*, from the Italian words *pelle agra*, meaning rough or painful skin. *Pellagra* it has been called ever since.

Unfortunately, treatment and understanding of the disease were not as successful as its naming. Suggested explanations for pellagra were legion. Breathing foul or humid air; contact with infected sheep, which seemed to suffer a similar disorder; heredity; a form of sunstroke; and a type of leprosy were all put forth at one time or another. Some observers, notably the great German writer and thinker Goethe, thought that faulty diet was the cause, for only poor people came down with the disease. He theorized that low-quality food, which was all the impoverished could afford, was responsible.

Corn bore the brunt of this indictment, since pellagra occurred most frequently among peasants who ate maize—the European name for corn—as the staple of their diet. Some felt unripe corn was the culprit; others, overripe. Most thought it was corn infected with a harmful microbe. One patriot even went so far as to accuse corn from America as the villain. Healthy European corn, he argued, could not possibly induce pellagra.

Cures were as bizarre as the proffered causes. Many were tried, with small doses of arsenic becoming the favorite. This poison only sped the victims to their deaths.

The debate over cause and cure rolled on for decades, through the nineteenth century and into the twentieth, while the death toll in Europe from pellagra mounted higher and higher.

Then the scene shifted to another continent. In 1907, a strange disease swept the Mount Vernon Insane Hospital in Alabama. Eighty-seven inmates endured weakness, diarrhea, rashes, and new forms of mental derangement. Fifty-seven of them died.

The calamity was diagnosed as the sickness of the four D's: dermatitis (skin rash), diarrhea, dementia (madness), and death. Pellagra had come to this country.

It spread with a vengeance, ascending swiftly to become a health problem of major proportions in the southern United States. In South Carolina it was the second leading cause of death. State and national conferences and commissions were called to combat the epidemic, with no result other than the advancement of more exotic causes and cures of little help. By 1915, there were over 100,000 cases of pellagra in the United States, with more than 10,000 people a year dying from the disease.

The situation grew desperate. Members of Congress urged the Surgeon General of the United States to take action.

In response to their outcry, the chief medical officer of the nation appointed Joseph Goldberger to head the U.S. Public Health Service's investigation into pellagra.

Goldberger, a naturalized American born in Hungary, was the ideal choice. At one time rejected by the U.S. Navy because he was a Jew, he had instead turned his talents to the field of medical research—with great success in the service of his adopted country. Tireless, courageous, and as logical as any Sherlock Holmes, he possessed the knack for pinning down the carriers of disease, as he showed when the skin eruptions of Schamberg's disease appeared among dock workers in Philadelphia. Called in to solve the problem, Goldberger discovered all the men affected had handled straw mattresses prior to the outbreak, and with further investigation he traced the straw to a single source in New Jersey.

Was this the answer?

To find out, he plunged his hand into a batch of straw and left it there for an hour. Less than a day later, the telltale sores blossomed. He had volunteers sleep on the suspected mattresses, and they, too, came down with the sickness. Careful sifting of the straw produced tiny mites, and those mites, when placed on the skin of another volunteer, produced more eruptions. Goldberger had tracked Schamberg's disease to its source.

He had similar success with Mexican typhus fever. Through a chain of brilliant logical deductions, he identified the body louse as the carrier, eliminating all other possibilities one by one.

Now, fresh from these triumphs, and from work on yellow fever, typhoid, and diphtheria, he closed grips with pellagra, a disease which had baffled and decimated mankind for almost two centuries.

Unlike many of his colleagues, Goldberger was not content to stay at home and theorize. Immediately upon his appointment he left Washington, D.C. to journey throughout the South, viewing the situation first hand and gathering clues to solve the scientific mystery.

He discovered that pellagra was rampant among the inmates of institutions which housed the debilitated and the insane; but he found not a single case of the disease among the doctors, nurses, or attendants working in these asylums. Surely, he thought, if pellagra were communicable, at least one instance of it should turn up among persons in daily contact with the afflicted. But none did. Also, in his travels, he found that the malady affected the poor exclusively, and not the middle class or the rich.

What could account for these facts?

To Goldberger, after close scrutiny, they suggested only one explanation: pellagra was induced by a *defective diet*, and not by germs or any of the other speculative causes advanced in the past, except this one, first espoused by Goethe. Quite simply, the medical personnel did not contract pellagra because they ate better food by taking the top-quality items for themselves and leaving the rest to the inmates. The staffers could also buy their food, and often did, outside the institutions—something the confined could not do, of course. As for poor people, Goldberger found they ate mostly bread, cereals, corn, and other vegetables, because they could not afford the expense of meat, milk, and eggs. He reasoned that some essential nutrient must be missing from the diets of the inmates and the impoverished, and that the lack of it impeded normal processes of the body, producing the effects called pellagra. In other words, he argued, pellagra was not a communicable sickness but a *deficiency* disease, the deficiency wreaking havoc on body chemistry.

Goldberger further surmised that the missing nutrient might be a vitamin, a new concept in the early 1900s. Corn? The public-health official concluded that there was nothing intrinsically wrong with this vegetable, that it was a good food, but that people should not build their entire diets around it, because corn lacked the nutrient that prevented pellagra. Eat a well-balanced diet, he advised, and pellagra would be averted.

Because his results were so radical, Goldberger and his findings quickly provoked entrenched and sometimes turbulent opposition from professional ranks. Louis Pasteur's theory that disease is produced by microbes had just finished its long, hard battle for acceptance by physicians and scientists. And now Goldberger wanted to upset the medical applecart by proclaiming that pellagra, one of the worst ravagers, was not caused by germs, but simply by eating too little of the right foods. How dare he! His critics demanded proof.

In a dramatic experiment, Goldberger gave them the final evidence. He assembled sixteen volunteers, swabbed their throats with saliva, and injected blood into them, both substances first extracted from pellagra victims. The volunteers then ate flour balls containing urine, nasal secretions, skin scrapings, and feces from people felled by the disorder under study. Some of the participants were nauseated by this mixture, but none came down with pellagra, thus proving it was not an infectious disease.

At the time of his report Goldberger did not name the brave volunteers working with him to expose the truth about pellagra. Today, their identities are known. Among them were Dr. and Mrs. Joseph Goldberger.

Other experiments soon followed, establishing that pellagra was induced by poor diet alone. Further research demonstrated that all but the most hopeless cases of this disease could be cured by eating foods rich in the unspecified nutrient.

Not satisfied to rest with revolutionary work well done, Goldberger took up the trail of this strange nutrient, the p-p (pellagra-preventing) factor, as he called it. Alas, the crowning glory of finding the p-p factor was not to be his. Goldberger died of cancer in 1929 before he could identify it.

In 1937 its discovery was finally announced; and, as he had believed, it was a vitamin. This missing nutrient was now called *niacin,* and it is a deficiency of niacin that causes pellagra.

Today, thanks to the beginnings made by Goldberger, pellagra has been so thoroughly conquered that most doctors in this country have never seen a case of it, and chances are they never will.

Yet the name Joseph Goldberger, unlike the name of Walter Reed, or that of Jonas Salk, is unknown to the general public, and to most people dreaded pellagra, one of the great destroyers of all time, is only a word seen briefly in textbooks and then quickly forgotten.

But the legacy of Goldberger and his work lives on.

THE DISCOVERY OF VITAMINS

The point of the foregoing story is not that you're in imminent danger of contracting pellagra if you diet or if you don't consume meat and eggs, but to impress upon you that there's so much more to eating and dieting than a discussion of calories, carbohydrates, protein, or fat. Anyone or any weight-reducing plan that talks exclusively of these subjects performs a strong disservice and is neglecting some basic components of your diet: vitamins and minerals. And they are the most vital part.

Calories, units measuring the energy value of foods, can come from carbohydrates, protein, or fat, which are present in any food; but the lack of one vitamin in your diet from eating the wrong foods, as Goldberger demonstrated, can cripple you, send you to the madhouse, or even kill you. The same is true of certain minerals. Do you see their relative importance?

The idea there were such substances in food necessary for good health did not really take hold until the early part of the twentieth century. Goldberger was one of the pioneers, although James Lind in his study of scurvy first glanced near the truth in the 1700s, as we shall see in Chapter Four.

This realization—that there are essential nutrients in foods—generated a flurry of research aimed at isolating the new substances and learning their functions in body chemistry. It also necessitated a label for them. In 1912, Casimir Funk, a Polish scientist working in London, suggested the name *vitamine*, from the Latin word *vita*, meaning "life," and *amine*, a chemical term denoting compounds of ammonia (vitamins were then believed to be related to this compound). The name Funk offered was accepted by the scientific community, and later the final *e* was dropped to form the word *vitamin* when it was learned the substances had little to do with ammonia or amines.

Years of toil by scientists passed before the first vitamin was isolated. Until that time vitamins were treated with awe and mystery, and some people doubted whether anything would be found.

But the tiny white crystals of thiamin detected in 1926 forever put an end to this speculation. Their discovery also explained in part the elusiveness of vitamins: they exist in food in very small quantities. A week's supply of thiamin for one person can be placed on the head of a pin.

THE ROLE OF VITAMINS

What are vitamins? And what do they do?

The first question is the more easily answered. Vitamins are organic compounds (chemical substances that contain carbon) which are not proteins, fats, or carbohydrates, and which have no caloric value in themselves. They're present in food in very small amounts and are necessary for growth in tissues, resistance to infection, utilization of food, normal reproduction, and overall good health. If they sound indispensable to you, you're right. We can't be without them.

Vitamins in their pure form are tiny, usually colorless crystals, not very different from table salt in appearance. A few are tinged with color. Riboflavin, a vitamin found abundantly in milk, has a somewhat orangeish tint.

The total number of recognized vitamins is fourteen.

Ten of them are water-soluble—that is, if stirred in water, they dissolve, again like table salt. Thiamin, riboflavin, niacin, biotin, choline, folacin, pantothenic acid, vitamin B-6, vitamin B-12, and vitamin C fall into this category. The remaining four vitamins, A, D, E, and K, are fat-soluble, meaning, for one thing, they're found only in fats and oils, a good reason to include some fats and oils in your diet. More about this later.

Keeping track of the number of vitamins can be confusing because researchers over the years have changed the names and numbers of these nutrients as more were discovered and as their chemical natures were revealed. For example, thiamin was first called vitamin B and then B_2 by the British, vitamin G by the Americans, and then B_1, B-1, thiamine, and finally thiamin, as it is known today.

Food faddists further cloud the issue. The faddists, who lay claim to more nutritional wisdom than Ph.D. nutritionists in universities and government, enthusiastically proclaim the presence of vitamin P, vitamin B-17, and so forth. Actually, the fourteen I have named are the only ones known, and the likelihood that more vitamins of major importance will be discovered is now remote.

There are a few nutrients that, for one technical reason or another, are not called vitamins. These substances, such as bioflavinoids, are required for the maintenance of good health, but because they're necessary in such small measure and are found in nearly every food, we can dispense with discussion of them and you need not worry about getting the proper amounts. More than sufficient quantities come from normal eating habits.

The answer to the second question, about the function of vitamins, is a bit more complex.

To explore it, let's look at the human body through the cold eyes of that most heartless person, the chemist. To him, and for the moment, to us, the body is a bag of chemicals, chemicals that constantly react with one another; this continuing interaction of elements and compounds keeps us alive. Observing the body from this viewpoint, we see, for example, oxygen combining with complicated molecules to produce energy; we find little molecules linking up to make bigger ones, and these joining and interlocking to create cells, which eventually form tissues and organs; and we see thousands of other reactions, all meshing together to complete the essential life processes.

Now, not all of these responses can happen by themselves. It's not like dumping Alka-Seltzer in a glass of water and watching it fizz. Sometimes the chemicals will just sit there. They need help to react, and this is where vitamins come in. The vitamins act as catalysts, or aids, to make the reaction go, themselves emerging unchanged at the end of the operation.

You can see a catalyst at work by pouring some powdered charcoal into a glass of hydrogen peroxide, the liquid used for bleaching and antiseptic purposes. The peroxide, quiet before the addition of the powder, boils and bubbles when the charcoal hits it, turning into plain water, oxygen frothing into the air. Nothing would have happened unless the catalyst had been added; but the black powder, though it triggers and participates in the reaction, comes out unchanged at the finish.

The same is true of vitamins. If an essential one isn't present, a needed process in the body won't take place. And when it doesn't, other procedures collapse, things go haywire inside you, and you develop what is called a deficiency disease. We already know about the relation of niacin to pellagra. There are others. Lack thiamin and your nerves won't function correctly; this condition is called beri-beri. Short on vitamin C? Your gums and skin start to rot, and you've fallen victim to scurvy.

Their catalytic quality makes vitamins necessary to good health. Unlike the charcoal in our example, however, these nutrients eventually break down, or are lost, and they have to be replaced in just the right amounts—not too much, not too little. This can be tricky, especially when you are on a weight-reducing diet.

We'll look at this problem and all the vitamins in succeeding chapters. You must know about them in order to diet properly. You don't want to replace the dangers of obesity with troubles arising from poor nutrition or vitamin overdosage, conditions more common than you might think.

MINERALS

Most of us have a better idea of what minerals are than we have of vitamins: minerals are inorganic substances (they lack carbon) like the metals, and sulfur and phosphorus. Though dissimilar to vitamins in make up, minerals, too, in minute amounts, play vital roles in the life processes. Iron, for instance, composes part of the material called hemoglobin that carries oxygen in the blood to all the cells. Calcium makes strong bones and teeth, as we remember from our school lessons, and sodium helps keep acids and alkalis in balance, something we may not have learned. We'll look at these and others in the following pages.

But first I want to say a few words on an important topic.

HOW MUCH IS ENOUGH?

Years upon years of inquiry and study by hundreds of scientists in scores of research institutions have given us an exact answer concerning this question about the proper amounts of vitamins and minerals needed by the human body. The answer comes in two stages.

Just to get by, we talk about the Minimum Daily Requirements, abbreviated MDR, a standard set by the Food and Drug Administration of the federal government. But ingest quantities of nutrients at the MDR level each day and you court deficiency diseases, for the MDR represents borderline amounts. Yet, until recently, cereal manufacturers delighted in apprising potential customers of how their products met these "government requirements," by containing, for instance, 10 milligrams of iron, the MDR for this mineral.

But times have changed; and the MDR is not for us.

We want something more, a standard that tells us there's no question we're getting enough, and yet not too much, for it's as possible to harm your health by ingesting excessive amounts of certain vitamins and minerals as it is to take in too little.

The criteria we seek are found in the Recommended Dietary Allowances, abbreviated RDA, the nutritional yardstick formulated by the Food and Nutrition Board of the National Academy of Sciences. The Board, a group of prestigious scientists, studies all available technical research on vitamins and minerals and, equipped with this information, prepares the RDA, revising the standard every four or five years to accommodate new advances.

The U.S. RDA, found on the nutrition labels of food, are values set by the Food and Drug Administration and are based largely on the 1968 RDA standards established by the Food and Nutrition Board of the National Academy of Sciences. The updated 1974 RDA are used in this book.

For each vitamin and mineral, the RDA gives the amount required daily to maintain perfect nutritional health. These levels cover almost everyone in the United States. The only exceptions are persons with severe medical or emotional problems—those who are under a doctor's care, or should be.

The amounts fixed by the Board are not minimums to ward off deficiency diseases. The quantities advocated in the RDA are designed to insure the best possible nutrition, while reflecting the differing needs of the American public with respect to sex, age, height, and weight. The demands of a twenty-year-old woman, for example, who is five feet, five inches tall and weights 128 pounds, are adequately served. For her, the RDA advises 18 milligrams (mg.) of iron a day, nearly twice the MDR for this mineral. So, unless you're physically ill or under abnormal emotional stress, the RDA embraces your nutritional requirements, plus a margin of safety, though without swinging into the dangers of overdosage.

Unfortunately, a surprising number of Americans are not at RDA levels at all, and poor nutrition, cutting across all social classes, is recognized as one of the biggest health problems in the country, possibly rivaling obesity itself. Government studies show that more than half the people in the United States fall below RDA requisites for thiamin, vitamin C, and calcium. In 1955 half the families surveyed met the federal definition of a good diet, with 15 percent falling into the poor category. Again in 1965 about 50 percent of the families interviewed rated good, but the number of people with poor diets had risen to 21 percent.

Today, the trend toward nutritional bankruptcy is accelerating.

Up to this point we've been talking about the population as a whole. Let's break the picture down a little.

Of the two sexes, women are hardest hit.

A recent study revealed that iron intake among females aged nine to fifty-four years falls 30 percent below the RDA level for that mineral, a staggering figure for those of us who know that iron is needed to prevent anemia. And the women fare worse than the men for nearly every other nutrient.

For the person on a weight-reducing diet, the situation deteriorates. More than half the people in this country, while eating too many calories, still do not get enough vitamins and minerals. Their bodies operate at less than peak efficiency. And when one of them cuts down on the amount of food he eats, hoping to lose weight, he unbalances his nutrition even further and courts problems as serious as those that accompany obesity. So serious, in fact, that the results can be—and have been—death.

In 1971, a twenty-four-year-old New Jersey woman who followed the Zen Macrobiotic Diet for nine months died from its effects—extreme malnutrition. And there has been a report of at least one other succumbing to a similar fate after going on this brown rice and tea diet.

Dieters might be excused for their ignorance, but not those who profess themselves experts and publish systems that claim to be the final solution to the weight-reduction problem.

These popular diet plans, which thousands follow, rarely take into account the necessity of total nutrition, and if they do, they pass quickly over it with the advice to take vitamin pills, a highly questionable practice, and one that can lead to effects as harrowing as those of any deficiency disease, as we shall see in the chapters ahead.

As a dieter, you certainly don't want part of one extreme or the other—too much nutrition or too little. Clearly, what you need is a diet plan that allows you to shed undesired pounds while meeting or exceeding the RDA levels of essential nutrients but without going overboard. Further, the diet plan should cater to normal tastes and eating patterns, should use regular food and not require supplements, and should permit you a great variety in food and meal selection.

And that is exactly what I provide you in this book—a safe, sensible way to diet.

Chapters Fifteen and Sixteen will tell you how to reduce the natural vitamin way, but before that let's look at the nutrients whose functions are most imperiled by dieting and the health and appearance problems that a reducing regimen might trigger.

3

VITAMIN A:
THE VISIBLE VITAMIN

THE KID-GLOVES NUTRIENT

Any diet plan you follow should provide adequate amounts of vitamin A. Without it you will suffer blindness, the ravages of disease, and even death. But your diet plan should not supply you with too much vitamin A, because in large quantities it becomes a terrible poison, causing bone deterioration, intense pain, and in extreme cases, possible death.

A necessary nutrient, vitamin A must be handled with care.

CHARACTERISTICS

Discovered in 1913, vitamin A is in reality several different molecules with similar properties which have "vitamin A" activity. One of these is an alcohol called retinol, the most potent form of the nutrient.

Vitamin A crystals are yellow in color and do not dissolve in water, but are soluble in fats, such as animal fat and butter.

Curiously, there are substances found abundantly in nature which are chemically just a step away from being vitamin A. These are the *carotenes* and a substance called *cryptoxanthin*. A molecule of carotene or cryptoxanthin can be split rather inefficiently into two molecules of vitamin A in the human body.

The carotenes are orangeish-yellow and give that color to carrots (where carotenes get their name), pumpkins, melons, peaches, and sweet potatoes. Cryptoxanthin lends its color to yellow corn. Hence, in contrast to most foods and their nutrients, you can actually see the potential vitamin these vegetables offer.

Yellow and orange vegetables are not the only sources of vitamin A. Dark-green vegetables like spinach, collards, and dandelion greens are also good. Carotene is present in them—its color is simply masked by the stronger green of chlorophyll.

The best food source for vitamin A, however, is liver. Vitamin A is stored in the liver of animals to be used when little is coming in through food—thus, the concentration of it in this organ. Beef liver is an excellent source of vitamin A, as are fish livers. Cod-liver oil is particularly rich in this vitamin.

Unlike some nutrients, vitamin A is not destroyed when you cook the foods that contain it. Nor is it soluble in water, so none is lost when the cooking water is thrown out—a hazard faced in the preparation of foods with water-soluble vitamins. Evaporation or pasteurization of milk does not eliminate much of this nutrient, either.

Vitamin A does have three weak points, however. One is exposure to air. Oxidation hastens the destruction of this vitamin. When butter turns rancid (oxidizes) or when vegetables dry out, vitamin A is lost. The second shortcoming is its response to light exposure. Ultraviolet light destroys this vitamin. For this reason, food containing vitamin A should be stored in a cold dark place, such as a refrigerator. The third drawback when dealing with vitamin A is that sometimes it is processed out of foods that would otherwise naturally contain it. So watch out for this problem. On occasion, however, vitamin A is added back into some foods or is put into foods that would not ordinarily offer it—for instance, cereals and margarines.

THE WORK OF VITAMIN A

Vitamin A plays an important part in many body functions. One of them is vision. Vitamin A is a component of visual purple, a pigment found in the retina of the eye. When light strikes the retina, the visual purple changes into another pigment called visual yellow. This metamorphosis sends nerve impulses to the brain, resulting in a "seeing" of the image falling on the back of the eyeball. In the dark the visual yellow turns back into visual purple.

But the process is not 100 percent efficient, and a small amount of visual purple is always lost in the transformation. Thus, it must constantly be renewed—from a steady supply of vitamin A. When this nutrient is not present, vision is impaired, and night blindness occurs, one of the first signs of vitamin A deficiency. In fact, the quickness of the eyes' ability to adapt to darkness is sometimes used to measure the supply of vitamin A in a person's body. (A point to note: though lack of vitamin A definitely causes night blindness, not all night blindness is caused by a dearth of vitamin A.)

Vitamin A is also required for the formation of mucopolysaccharides, molecules that are essential components of mucous membranes. If vitamin A is unavailable, the mucous membranes deteriorate; and the epithelial cells, cells which line parts of the body exposed to the environment—such as the skin and the linings of the throat, lungs, and intestines—lose their integrity, drying up, thereby leaving the body vulnerable to attack by bacteria. The first indications, then, of vitamin A deficiency (besides night blindness) are dry skin, sore throat, sinus trouble, dry eyes, and poor hearing. As the bacterial invasion mounts, abscesses of the mouth and ears may develop, and the eyes may become infected, leading to a blinding disease called xerophthalmia. The skin will take on an ugly, scaly appearance, with horny material clustered at the base of each hair follicle. Moreover, bacteria may enter through the stomach and intestines and spread disease throughout the entire body. The lungs will become predisposed toward tuberculosis.

Vitamin A is also necessary for the proper formation of bones and teeth. They will not grow right without it. For instance, during childhood the cranium may enlarge too slowly for the rapidly expanding brain and cause pressure on this organ, and cavities will develop in teeth.

Vitamin A is essential for normal reproduction. Lack of it can cause sterility or miscarriage. In rats, the males become sterile, and in pregnant females the embryo resorbs into the uterus.

The ultimate outcome of vitamin A deficiency is death.

EXTENT OF DEFICIENCY

Sadly, vitamin A deficiency (technically called avitaminosis or hypovitaminosis A) is all too prevalent in the world. Along with protein deficiency, called kwashiorkor, vitamin A deficiency is the most common form of malnutrition found in the underdeveloped countries.

Children are the hardest hit in these places. A hospital in Java reports that over 80 percent of its blindness cases in children under ten years of age stems from vitamin A deficiency. Throughout the world, it annually blinds close to 100,000 children, many of whom subsequently die.

The picture is different in the United States. Most people here receive enough vitamin A from their diet, so vitamin A deficiency is rare in this country. However, the intake for certain groups of women, adolescents and elderly women, appears to be marginal. And according to national surveys, average intake of vitamin A by all of us has decreased in recent years. The figure now hovers just above the RDA.

Dieting, by affecting food and nutrient supply to the body, can only make the situation more precarious. A fad diet that concentrates on a few foods that might lack vitamin A can be especially dangerous.

PILLS

But don't run out and stock up on vitamin pills to insure that you're getting enough vitamin A as you diet. People who take these pills are often unknowingly gambling with their health, because some who take them operate on what may be called the "more is better" theory. Expanded, it reads like this: "If a little of something is good for you, then more of it must be better yet." In this case they would say that since a small amount of vitamin A is good for you (preventing the horrors of deficiency), then a lot of vitamin A must be very good for you (better eyesight, etc.). Consequently, they take massive doses of it through pills.

But the theory is unsound, and the practice of taking pills as supplements dangerous.

For example, ingesting large doses of thiamin, a water-soluble vitamin, is harmless; but neither does it promote increased health in any way. On the other hand, large does of niacin, another water-soluble vitamin, can cause flushing of the face, dizziness, and a feeling of heat and itching. Several hundred times the RDA of niacin can induce diarrhea, nausea, and vomiting. Fortunately, the deleterious effects of excessive amounts of the water-soluble vitamins such as thiamin and niacin are generally minimal, since much of the excess is excreted in the urine. However, the same cannot be said of the fat-soluble vitamins.

Vitamin A is one of these, not soluble in water, so inordinate amounts are not excreted in the urine. Instead, vitamin A is stored in the liver until it breaks down in time under the natural processes of degradation. But huge quantities can accumulate in this organ—and they can be toxic.

The August 24, 1961, issue of the New England Journal of Medicine reports the case of a thirty-two-year-old homemaker who had been taking 100,000 International Units (IU) daily of vitamin A (25 times the RDA) via pills for over two years. She complained of fatigue, nausea, and falling hair. Also, she felt pain in her back, right hip, and abdomen. She was listless and displayed little interest in her activities. Her doctor diagnosed her condition as vitamin A overdosage. All of her symptoms disappeared when she stopped her vitamin A intake.

Strangely, vitamin overdose can give rise to many of the same effects of vitamin deficiency, the very troubles that in normal amounts they prevent. Vitamin A is an example in point. As we have seen, this nutrient is necessary for proper bone growth in children. Too little can produce deformity—but so can too much. Several case histories of hypervitaminosis A (vitamin A overdose) reported in the December 8, 1962, issue of the Journal of the American Medical Association reveal instances of resulting bone damage. Here, children were fed massive doses of vitamin A for "insurance" by their mothers. These unfortunate children had one leg develop shorter than the other and felt pain on walking. One three-year-old girl refused to walk at all because the pain was so intense. She grew up with her left leg almost two inches shorter than her right. Deplorably, these effects are not reversible.

Beyond the chance of overdosage there is another danger to vitamin pills. Believe it or not, you can still incur vitamin deficiency while taking pills as a form of insurance, because vitamin pills do not generally include all the needed nutrients. So if your eating patterns do not produce enough of a certain nutrient, and the pill you rely on also does not contain this nutrient, unknowingly you will become the victim of a deficiency.

For instance, one popular brand of vitamin pill includes vitamins A, D, C, B-6, B-12, thiamin, riboflavin, niacin, pantothenic acid, and iron. You may take this pill, believing you are safe from any nutritional inadequacy. But this product lacks folacin. And if your diet is also short on folacin (easily accomplished by shunning green vegetables, which many people do), you will contract a form of anemia and soon feel sluggish and tired. This same popular brand does not contain calcium, though calcium deficiency is a serious problem in the United States. Neither does it have in its composition the small amounts of other vitamins and minerals whose consumption is obligatory to life and health.

CONCLUSION

What does all this mean? That you should forsake thoughts of vitamin A and the other nutrients as you reduce, fiddling with foods and diets while you ignore the dangers of deficiency? Or that you should take pills and risk overdosage with no real assurance that you're actually avoiding deficiency?

No, none of these alternatives.

It means that for vitamin A and the other nutrients there is a certain range of intake, centered around the RDA, that you must have for normal body functioning and good health.

And that the RDA is best obtained by eating regular food. Pills contain only what's been put into them—but a wise selection of food covers the whole spectrum of nutrients, whether they're well-known, obscure, or undiscovered.

Normal food can supply all the nutrition you need; and in addition, when you depend on food and not pills for your vitamins and minerals, not only do you receive everything you require, you also raise a natural barrier against vitamin overdosage, a protection vitamin pills cannot provide. Natural foods, because of the impossibly large quantities you would have to eat, will not poison you with too much nutrition.

So the RDA and normal foods both represent built-in nutritional insurance, the RDA against deficiency, and regular foods against vitamin overdosage.

There is only one difficulty: as you diet, RDA standards are harder to achieve, because you're altering the kinds and amounts of food you eat.

But if you follow the diet plans in this book, you do not have to worry.

Scientific construction of the plans, with the help of a high speed modern digital electronic computer, has taken care of not only reducing and calorie considerations, but the RDA requirements as well, including those of nutrients like vitamin A, agents which must be treated with caution.

4

VITAMIN C: SUPERVITAMIN?

"BLACKENED GUMS AND FALLING TEETH"

Vitamin C is integral to life.

Deprived of it, you'd die a horrible, stinking death—your teeth falling from gangrenous gums, your flesh rotting on bones too brittle to support your weight. This is death from scurvy. It has raised a lot of tombstones through history.

Scurvy swept through the warriors of the Seventh Crusade. Jean, Sire de Joinville—knight and boon companion to Saint Louis, King of France and leader of the crusade in thirteenth-century Egypt—describes the catastrophe:

> . . . there came upon us the sickness of the host, which sickness was such that the flesh of our legs dried up, and the skin upon our legs became spotted, black and earth color, like an old boot; and with us, who had the sickness, the flesh of our gums putrefied; nor could anyone escape from this sickness, but he had to die. The sign of death was this, that when there was bleeding from the nose, then death was sure.
>
> . . . The sickness began to increase in the host in such sort, and the dead flesh so to grow upon the gums of our people, that the barber surgeons had to remove the dead flesh in order

that the people might masticate their food and swallow it. Great pity it was to hear the cry throughout the camp of the people whose dead flesh was being cut away; for they cried like women laboring of child.

The crusade had gone badly. The Moslems severed the Europeans' supply line halfway along the march to Cairo, encircled their enemy, and settled in for a long siege, content with slowly starving the Christian invaders to death. It was then the disease struck. Scurvy. And Joinville gives us a perfect portrayal of its harrowing effects—the deterioration and putrefaction of the body—now known to be induced by a deficiency of vitamin C.

Joinville himself survived its ravages, was captured by the Saracens, and was later ransomed with Saint Louis and set free. The other poor victims of the blight, both the dead and the dying, were burned by the Moslems in a great fire with their weapons and war machines.

Neither the Saracens nor anyone else back then understood the origin of scurvy, though the affliction had been long known to the world. The first description of scurvy dates back nearly 3500 years and comes from the Chinese. A millennium after that, Hippocrates listed the symptoms as they afflicted Greek soldiers about 400 B.C.: the pains in the legs, the blackened gums, the falling teeth. This is scurvy's familiar pattern, woven again and again down through the centuries. But cause, correction, and prevention remained obscure. Ignorance and scurvy raged on. So badly did it decimate the population of Europe in the fifteenth and sixteenth centuries, the horrified doctors of the period thought all diseases might derive from it.

The curse was especially prevalent among crews of ships making long ocean crossings. Vasco da Gama lost over half his nautical company to scurvy when he rounded Africa and the Cape of Good Hope in 1498. Magellan's ship circumnavigated the globe in 1522, a great feat. But the men aboard paid the price, the majority falling to scurvy by the end of the historic voyage. Magellan himself fell to an attack by cannibals, a calamity of a different sort—unlucky, but not widespread.

In the next two hundred years more and more sailors dropped to the deck with the odious symptoms. By the eighteenth century, scurvy had claimed a greater number of lives in the British navy than had enemy action.

Something had to be done.

Sailors and scurvy—an abhorrent by-product of the Age of Discovery—would be the clue that led to the cure.

PULLING THE CLAWS OF THE MONSTER

James Lind, A Scottish surgeon in the British Royal Navy, wanting to eradicate scurvy from the seas, in the 1700s studied the affliction first hand and from ships' reports.

His most intriguing bit of information was a story about a crewman who fell ill to scurvy and was put ashore on Greenland—which happened to be nearby—to keep the disease from spreading to his companions and to fend for himself. The man didn't die but survived, so the account went, by eating grass and roots. And his case of scurvy vanished. The man hailed a passing ship and made his way home.

Lind thought over the puzzling and unlikely narrative. What if it were true? Could scurvy then be cured by a change in eating habits? It was worth finding out.

Expectantly, the good doctor went among his patients, handing out experimental diets. Most proved ineffective. Drinking and soaking food in vinegar didn't work. But sucking lemons and oranges did.

Lind soon found that eating citrus fruits in general cured scurvy. And he felt ingesting them might be a good preventive measure. The doctor published his results in 1753 under the title, "A Treatise on Scurvy," and never did a piece of scientific literature make a smaller splash. But that's a fate unfortunately common to many a great work at the time of its introduction.

One of the few who did more than yawn was Captain James Cook, the great explorer. "Eat fruits and vegetables," he cried to his men, "and ward off scurvy on these long voyages of discovery to the Pacific." The crew looked up at their captain askance, shook their heads at the man who obviously had stood too long in the sun without his hat, and went right on with their grog and salted meat.

Cook performed an excessive amount of head scratching and came up with an idea. The next time he and his fellow officers sat down for a meal, they pretended to heartily enjoy eating the sauerkraut and the other less appetizing vegetables on their plates. The men serving them rushed back to their fellows and angrily reported that the officers were hogging one of the greater pleasures of the cruise—vegetables. Soon the entire crew clamored for equal treatment and victuals, and Cook, leaving scurvy behind, sailed on to the sound of munching, to bump into Australia.

News of Lind's cure finally worked its way up to top naval brass, and in 1795 they issued orders requiring each ship to carry some form of citrus fruit, and in particular, lime juice, because it didn't spoil like the fresh fruit from which it was squeezed.

And so, as every junior-high-school student can tell you, the British sailors, cured of scurvy but with puckered mouths, went on to be called "limeys" forevermore; and today by extension all Britons are nicknamed limey—an appellation, by the way, at which they take no offense.

Gradually, as knowledge spread of the curing power of fruits and vegetables, the signs of scurvy disappeared from the high seas and from many parts of the world.

A few years ago, modern scientists desiring to make an up-to-date study of the disease reproduced the ancient symptoms not in sailors, but in prisoner volunteers of the Iowa State Penitentiary. They did this by giving the inmates a diet lacking in vitamin C but sufficient in all the other nutrients.

The researchers noted few ill effects until the first month had passed. Then the convicts' skins became dry, itchy, and rough. The hair on their bodies coiled up, and their eyes turned bloodshot. The men complained of fatigue and pain; and because of this they had to curtail their exercise program. Their mouths became dry, fillings in their teeth fell out, and they were plagued with cavities. Near the end of the study swollen and bleeding gums were common. Depression and personality changes appeared with the physical symptoms.

The experiment lasted three months. Not all of the convicts finished the study. Two of them escaped, and hopefully, like the man stranded on Greenland, somehow replenished their supply of the missing vitamin. To those who remained inside the walls, vitamin C was administered and, as is usual with deficiency diseases, the victims recovered completely, demonstrating the relationship of vitamin C to scurvy.

Had the study continued, the convicts' bones would have turned brittle; the men would have developed anemia and a weakening of the heart and muscle fibers; and if the experiment had been carried to its ultimate conclusion, the prisoners would have died.

THE CHARACTERISTICS OF VITAMIN C

Scientists, pressing hard to discover the identity of mysterious vitamins that averted deficiency diseases, in 1918 labeled the scurvy-preventing factor in food vitamin C. In 1928 vitamin C was isolated from fruit juices, and in 1933 it was synthesized from simple sugars and given the chemical name *ascorbic acid*, because of its anti-scurvy properties.

Ascorbic acid crystals are water-soluble, odorless, and colorless. The orange color of the tablets sold in health food stores and drug stores is added later.

How important is vitamin C? So important that it's found in every single cell of the human body. Yet in many ways vitamin C remains a mystery. We speak of this nutrient in generalities. We know that it's essential to good health and to life itself, but beyond that we know little. Scientists believe this vitamin may function as a carrier of hydrogen in the cells in much the same way that hemoglobin transports oxygen in the blood. It may also play a part in the manufacture of the crucial hemoglobin.

Vitamin C is necessary to form collagen, a protein which makes up cartilage, the substance that composes your nose bone and kneecaps and which serves as a cushion in the knee joints—where it gives football players occasional trouble.

Another role vitamin C seems to play is in the healing of wounds. A higher concentration of it is found at the site of a wound than in the surrounding tissues. And a wound won't mend properly if the body lacks the normal amount of this nutrient.

Scientists also recognize that vitamin C somehow guards against infection. People with low levels of it are more susceptible to illness than persons with the normal quantity in their systems.

This now brings us to two related and much-debated questions: How much vitamin C does the human body need, and do people in this country get enough of it?

Let me begin the discussion by asking you a riddle.

DEFICIENCY TO EXTRAVAGANCY

Here it is: what do apes, monkeys, guinea pigs, the fruit-eating bat, and the red-vented bulbul bird have in common with man?

Give up?

The answer is that all these creatures, like man, must extract the vitamin C they require from the food they eat, with the penalty of contracting scurvy if they don't. Other animals, like your dog or the finicky cat on the television commercials, manufacture the vitamin C they need right inside their bodies.

Sailors got scurvy, but the ships' rats never did.

Thus, man and the bulbul bird are handicapped, staying one step ahead of scurvy by reason of what they put into their mouths.

Today in the United States outright scurvy is extremely rare. But latent scurvy isn't. This condition results from near-minimal intakes of vitamin C and is characterized by fatigue, depression, swollen or painful joints, and black and blue spots on the skin. According to the National Nutrition Survey many people *do* have borderline intakes of vitamin C, and 10 to 30 percent of the population may be *below* marginal levels. Now if you couple this with the fact that the vitamin C intake per person is steadily dropping each year, then the health picture doesn't look good. Latent scurvy will be on the upswing.

People aren't eating right. And the plight can only be worse for dieters. They're cutting down on food from a diet already deficient!

Okay, you say, some people don't get enough vitamin C from their diet, especially when they're reducing. Then should they take pills? And how much *is* enough? And can too much be dangerous, as in the case of the fat-soluble vitamins?

We'll look at the second question first—the problem of sufficiency. Meticulous scientific research has established that the absolute minimum amount of vitamin C necessary to ward off scurvy for the average adult is 10 mg per day. Three times that amount, or 30 mg, promotes good health.

Now, after careful study of all research, the Food and Nutrition Board of the National Academy of Sciences specifies 45 mg a day as the Recommended Dietary Allowance for adults. The amount the Board has set is one-and-a-half times the quantity needed to maintain good health and insures against vitamin loss in the cooking and storage of foods. Remember, in arriving at this figure the scientists on the Board have no axes to grind, drums to beat, pills to push, or rent to pay on health-food stores. But they do take great pride in their quest for truth. So 45 mg of vitamin C a day is all you need; and you can get almost three times that amount by eating right—even while on a diet.

Then what about those who advocate taking 10, 50, even 100 or 250 times that amount every day through pills and the miracles ascribed to these massive doses; the prevention of colds and the promotion of well-being and heightened sexual activity?

The evidence to support such claims isn't persuasive.

Linus Pauling, the Nobel Prize-winning chemist, champions the heavy-dosage view for cold prevention and is largely responsible for the public's attention to vitamin C. But his belief is based largely on the statistics of two people—himself and his wife—and how vitamin C affected them. A sample population of two, as you might guess, is not very good statistics.

May I illustrate? I have two friends who take 1000 mg of vitamin C via pills every day. Last winter one friend caught two colds and the other came down with two colds and the flu. I myself didn't get a single cold and all my vitamin C comes from normal foods—about 120 mg a day. So much for the statistics of two or three.

Several years ago researchers carried out a study of a more scientific nature than mine or Pauling's on vitamin C and colds. The experiment involved 91 people. Forty-seven of them took pills containing 1000 mg of vitamin C each day, while the remaining 44 swallowed similar-looking pills containing a harmless and inert substance. Neither group knew which pill was which, so psychological influences were barred from the experiment.

At the end of three days the researchers injected everyone with cold viruses. The 91 people continued taking their pills for six more days. During that time *no* difference in severity or number of colds was noted between the two groups.

Another study involving 3000 mg per day produced similar results. Huge amounts of vitamin C had no effect on cold prevention or cure.

In fairness to Dr. Pauling and his adherents, there is some evidence that leans ever so slightly in the direction of his belief. But it's as easily explained as a statistical aberration as anything else. Now this experiment has been redone, and it shows vitamin C has no influence on colds.

At this point you might call to my attention that vitamin C is necessary to fight infection. That's right. But there's no proof that anything beyond the 30 milligrams needed for good health works any better at battling disease.

The same is true for claims of increased feelings of well-being and heightened sexual activity. No proof.

Then where do these assertions come from?

Some may arise because of the "placebo effect." As you might know, a placebo is medication given solely to satisfy a patient and has no medicinal value. For example, our neighbor Mrs. Malarkey trudges wearily in to see the family physician, Dr. Hypo. She raises her hand weakly and declares, "I've been feeling so tired and run-down these past weeks, Dr. Hypo. I think I must have some dread disease."

Dr. Hypo gives Mrs. Malarkey a thorough examination and finds nothing physically wrong with her. But from rumor he's heard that her husband has run away with an ex-Rockette, her son is home moping around the house because he was booted out of college again, her spayed dog had ten puppies, and she has yet to win anything in the state lottery. The doctor knows that what Mrs. Malarkey needs is a psychological boost.

"It's nothing to worry about," Dr. Hypo exclaims with a merry smile. "Just take one of these pills every four hours and you'll feel like new."

Mrs. Malarkey, being the good lady that she is, sighs in relief, does as her doctor tells her, and sure enough in a short time is feeling much better.

Of course, the pills contained only a little starch. But with unswerving faith in Dr. Hypo, she fooled herself into getting better. This is the placebo effect. Mrs. Malarkey knew the pills would do the trick, and if anyone were to ask her, they did.

The same may be true for vitamin C pills. If you really think lots of vitamin C will alleviate a cold, pep you up, or turn you into a rutting Don Juan, then it might well work that way. The placebo effect is well known and has been documented for vitamin C. Pauling himself was convinced to try massive doses by a friend who said they would perform wonders for him.

Placebos, in general, are harmless, but we're not as sure about the huge doses of vitamin C. Persons taking them at gram level or above for the first time may suffer from burning stomachs—it is ascorbic *acid*—and diarrhea. Long-term high levels may increase the chance of kidney-stone development and in pregnant women may upset the enzyme systems of the unborn child, subjecting it to scurvy at birth because of its adjustment to abnormal amounts. Other long-range effects are as yet unknown. We await studies in this area. Until then, be wary.

Another argument advanced against taking large quantities of vitamin C by the use of pills is that the same amounts of the vitamin are unavailable to man in regular food. Up to 1933, when the vitamin was first made artificially, man just couldn't get plus-gram levels into his system. At least archeologists have yet to turn up any vitamin C factories on the site of ancient Troy. So any amount ingested above that provided by normal eating habits would not be of any nutritional value. The effects would be pharmacological or medicinal in nature, and because of this, such high levels should be taken only under the supervision of a doctor.

I'd like to add an argument of my own against devouring large quantities of vitamin C—an economic one—cost. Scientists have discovered that most of any excess vitamin C consumed beyond that necessary for good health is excreted in the urine a few hours after ingestion.

In light of that, let's consider the following calculation.

Suppose you take 3 grams of vitamin C a day in the form of tablets, and as much as 100 mg of it—more than twice the RDA—is absorbed by your body. Now 3 grams is 3000 mg, so that 3000 minus 100, or 2900 mg, is excreted in your urine. If you spend $5.95 on a bottle of 250 vitamin C tablets, then $\frac{2900}{3000}$ × $5.95, or $5.77, is passed from your body, leaving you with only 18 cents worth of vitamin C for almost a six dollars' expenditure. This is equivalent to buying 15 gallons of gasoline for your car, keeping only two quarts of it, and pouring the rest down the drain. Hardly good economics.

Economics, of course, is only one factor in the overall vitamin C picture. We've also looked at scurvy, the functions of vitamin C, the necessary requirements, the deficiencies in some people, the excesses others go to with this nutrient, and the perils involved.

Putting it all together, I can come to only one conclusion—that it's best to get all the vitamin C we need from natural foods. That way, we run no dangers and we save money, two powerful considerations.

And you can get more than enough vitamin C from the foods you eat. You simply do this by selecting the right foods in the right quantities—something especially important if you're on a reducing diet when total calories also have to be reckoned with.

If you accept my conclusion about natural foods, and I hope you do, because it's a sensible one, then the next thing you'll want to know is which foods contain vitamin C, and how to keep calories to a minimum.

FOOD, DIETING, AND VITAMIN C

By far the best sources of vitamin C are fresh vegetables and fruits, and particularly citrus fruits—oranges, lemons, limes—and their juices. Strawberries and cantaloupes, too, are rich in this vitamin. So are other fresh fruits. Just page through the listings in the Appendix.

Some of the green vegetables are excellent sources. One stalk of fresh broccoli has 2.5 times more vitamin C than a fresh orange. Potatoes also are good.

Potatoes? you ask.

Ah, the much-maligned potato. I want to say a few words for it.

A baked potato contains one-third the daily Recommended Dietary Allowance for vitamin C. In the year 1900 potatoes and sweet potatoes supplied half of everyone's vitamin C requirement. But today, the potato has slipped, providing us with only one-fifth of our intake of this precious nutrient. Weight-conscious persons are eating less of them. They believe the potato to be fattening because of its carbohydrate content.

This belief is erroneous.

As we shall see, if you eat too much of *any* food, regardless of its carbohydrate content, you'll get fat. It's calories, not just carbohydrates, that count. In this respect a baked potato is less fattening than two ounces of chipped beef, which contains virtually no carbohydrates. A baked potato has 90 calories, while that little bit of chipped beef has 115 calories hidden in it.

The potato just doesn't deserve its bad reputation. In fact, the potato is a hero. Its discovery in the New World and its importation back to Europe wiped out those epidemics of scurvy in the fifteenth and sixteenth centuries that we spoke of earlier.

I've included this tuberous paladin in my diet plan, not because of its valor, but because of its high nutritional value. The next time you see a potato on your plate from one of my menus, you don't have to salute it, but don't hesitate to eat it. The potato tastes good, is relatively cheap, and has lots of vitamin C.

Now you ask: how do you maintain adequate levels of vitamin C while keeping the calories down?

Relax—the computer and I have done it for you. Just follow the diet plans in Chapters 15 and 16. The smallest amount of vitamin C you can get on one day of my diet plan is 60 milligrams. That's one and one-third times the RDA for this nutrient combined with a minimum number of energy units so you can take that excess weight off safely.

I'm not shortchanging you on vitamin C.

GETTING THE MOST VITAMIN C FOR YOUR MONEY

You can shortchange yourself in food preparation and cooking.

Vitamin C is the most fragile of all vitamins and is easily destroyed by oxidation and sunlight. Keep your fruits and vegetables in a cold place, preferably the refrigerator, and you'll maximize their vitamin C content.

When you prepare fruits and vegetables, take care not to bruise or rip them. Cut them cleanly with a knife. Bruising or ripping activates an enzyme which hastens oxidation and speeds vitamin C destruction. Since this enzyme is like a time bomb, you should eat vitamin C-rich foods shortly after preparation to keep to a minimum any loss caused by the release of this digestant.

Cooking with baking soda destroys vitamin C, as does cooking in copper ware if the copper is on the *inside* of the pot. Copper and vitamin C don't get along chemically. Copper on the outside *only* of the pot is okay.

These few precautions will help you get more vitamin C from your food.

Is vitamin C the supervitamin? It's certainly one of the main building blocks of life, and without it the structure of your body would quickly crumble and decay. However, vitamin C is not another penicillin or aureomycin. It has no infection-fighting capabilities beyond the small amount required for good health that's obtainable from a balanced diet. It's like the shingles on the roof of your house. Put on properly, one layer of shingles will keep out the rain as effectively as 2, 3 or 250 layers. Too many layers and the roof just might come tumbling in. So be circumspect.

And be careful not to ignore the next nutrient when you're reducing. It's a mineral, but it's as invaluable to your health as vitamin C. Turn the page and I'll tell you about iron.

5

IRON: DEFICIENCY OF
SLOW SUFFOCATION

THE BIG ONE

The greatest single nutritional problem in the United States today is iron deficiency.

Iron deficiency affects about one out of four people in this country, the large majority of them women. And yet it is one of the least-known problems in America. Beyond a few television commercials advertising preparations containing iron, we hear little about it. Nonetheless, this most widespread of deficiencies is a condition that can lead to an ailment of serious consequences, a type of anemia that slowly chokes the life from the body.

And the simple deficiency itself is a great robber of vitality.

As a difficulty that may be compounded by dieting, iron deficiency is worthy of a detailed examination.

AN OLD FRIENDSHIP

Iron is the familiar gray metal.

By weight, it is the most abundant element of the earth, constituting 35 percent of the planet, with the major portion located in pure form at the center of the globe. Iron at the earth's surface, making up 5 percent of the crust, is seldom found in the free state, however, because it so readily combines with oxygen, forming various oxides of the metal.

One of the most versatile of materials, used in everything from cooking pots to skyscrapers, iron has long been a work horse of man, its discovery lost in the mists of antiquity. Also known for centuries as a tonic for anemia, iron's role as a nutrient necessary to the human system was confirmed experimentally in the nineteenth century by a French chemist, Boussingault.

THE LIFE-BRINGER

The total amount of iron in the human body is small, about 3 or 4 grams, or about the weight and mass of a half-dozen paper clips. About 25 percent of this quantity is stored in the liver, spleen, and bone barrow. Another 5 percent or so is scattered throughout the various tissues, where it plays a role as an irreplaceable component of enzymes. But the bulk of iron in the body, about 70 percent, is found in the red blood cells—as the most vital part of hemoglobin, the protein which carries life-giving oxygen to every cell of the body via the bloodstream. Each hemoglobin molecule contains four atoms of iron.

Iron's association with hemoglobin is perhaps its most important contribution to the life processes. When we breathe in, red blood cells circulating through the vessels in the lungs pick up oxygen from the air inhaled. Passing into the cells, the oxygen atoms attach themselves to the atoms of iron in the hemoglobin of the corpuscles, turning the hemoglobin a bright red. (This process gives arterial blood its rich color.)

From the lungs, the red blood cells travel through the arteries to the capillaries, where they release their oxygen atoms to the tissues. The individual cells of the tissues use the oxygen in chemical reactions to maintain life. In exchange for the oxygen, the hemoglobin picks up carbon dioxide, a waste product of cellular functioning, and becomes darker red. (This is the process that lends veinous blood its deeper hue.) From the tissues the red cells flow back through the veins to the lungs and there yield their cargo of carbon dioxide, which is exhaled as we breathe out. When we breathe in again, the red cells that have just relinquished carbon dioxide take on oxygen, and the cycle repeats itself.

It is the ability of iron to combine with oxygen in this process that allows us to live. So the next time you see your lawn chairs rusting outside, don't curse the corrosion and wish that iron didn't rust—it's iron's affinity for oxygen that keeps us alive.

STOCKPILING

The human body hoards its store of iron as closely as any miser hoards his gold, so precious is iron to life.

It even resorts to recycling.

As red blood cells die (lifetime, 4 months) and can no longer carry oxygen and carbon dioxide, the iron in them is incorporated into new corpuscles manufactured in the bone marrow.

A minimal amount of iron does escape the body by natural means, however, through falling hair, trimming of nails, and perspiration. Some is also lost when skin cells are rubbed off the body and when cells of the intestinal wall are scraped away by the passage of food. Very little iron is excreted in the urine.

The body can lose a major amount of iron through a decrease in blood supply.

In females, the natural processes of menstruation and pregnancy take their tolls, with iron loss through the menses half again the quantity lost to hair, nails, and so forth. Pregnancy also makes high demands on iron, for the mother must share her stock with her unborn infant and must forfeit further iron when blood is lost at delivery.

Excessive iron loss can occur in either sex when blood supply is quickly or continuously reduced, such as from open wounds, bleeding ulcers, or hemorrhoids. Too-frequent blood donations can also deplete iron stores—a pint of blood contains 250 mg of iron, or 25 times the RDA for men. Though normal iron loss can be replaced by food ingestion, when these unusual blood-loss conditions transpire, the situation should be monitored by a doctor to determine whether iron supplements are needed as an additional source of iron.

IRON DEFICIENCY, DIETING, AND IRON POISONING

For many Americans, and particularly for women because of menstruation and pregnancy, the balance between iron intake and iron loss is quite precarious and can easily be tipped in the wrong direction.

What happens to a person when iron loss exceeds iron intake?

At first, the stores of iron the body keeps in the spleen and liver for pregnancies (in the case of women) and emergencies are drained. This iron is now used to make hemoglobin in an effort to maintain the number of red blood cells at the proper level, and in making the iron-containing enzymes. At this point, when iron stores are low or exhausted, the person affected is said to be *iron deficient.*

Once the iron stores are depleted, and the deficit between iron intake and loss persists, the amount of hemoglobin in the blood begins to fall, simply because there is not enough iron to hold it at optimum quantity. As a consequence, red blood cells become shrunken, and the tissues, without the hemoglobin to bring oxygen, commence to "strangle" from lack of this vital element. Life processes start to break down. The person involved has contracted *iron deficiency anemia.*

The first outward indications of anemia are feelings of sluggishness, fatigue, and perhaps poor appetite and constipation. The victim may also suffer apathy and mental depression. But since these symptoms are characteristic of any number of ailments, both physical and mental, they may go unrecognized as signs of iron deficiency anemia.

If the situation is not rectified and the anemia continues, the symptoms increase in severity; the victim may exhibit pallor of the skin, a shortness of breath, and he may become dizzy and subject to fainting.

These conditions are overt manifestations of too little hemoglobin. Lack of hemoglobin causes the skin to look pale in comparison to normal skin, the color of which is heightened by the red cast hemoglobin gives to blood in the tissues. The shortness of breath, dizziness, and fainting occur because the tissues are oxygen starved, presenting much the same effect as would breathing at high altitudes where the air is thin. Sleeping too much is a symptom of the general slowing of body functioning.

Death is the inevitable finish to iron deficiency anemia.

Fortunately, not many people in this country suffer this final stroke.

But the figures for iron deficiency in the United States are nonetheless staggering, with five million women estimated to be victims of iron deficiency anemia and another twenty-five million judged to be iron deficient. Most won't die—but many will labor under poor health, and some will experience real debilitating effects.

What makes the problem so great?

Excessive blood-loss conditions, such as bleeding ulcers and too-frequent blood donations, contribute; but the problem stems primarily from a lack of iron in the diet—an insufficient intake of this mineral through food ingestion.

A Department of Agriculture survey shows that while the typical male receives enough iron in his diet to enjoy good health, the average female, who requires nearly twice as much, does not. The eating habits of women aged twenty to fifty-four years produced only 70 percent or less of their RDA for iron daily. Girls from childhood age to adolescence also fell well below RDA standards. As the Food and Nutrition Board of the National Academy of Sciences has pointed out, the RDA of 18 mg of iron for adult women virtually cannot be met by the typical American diet.

This covers the population in general.

For dieters, prospects worsen.

Possibly already stumbling along the narrow ledge of iron deficiency, dieters, by decreasing or modifying their food intake, may plunge right over the brink into actual iron deficiency anemia—with all its concomitant medical problems.

We're talking about real people, remember, people like you who are contemplating weight reduction by dieting, and who unknowingly may compromise their health if they do not include enough iron in their reducing regimens.

But acquiring dietary iron takes a great deal of thought and planning. After all, ordinary people don't get enough iron in their diets. Is it possible for the dieter to overcome this obstacle?

Yes.

In fact, in the diet plans explained in Chapters Fifteen and Sixteen the work has been done for you. Along with a sensible weight loss, these plans will provide you with at least 18 mg of iron daily, the RDA for adult women, which is nearly twice that of men. What's more, the iron you'll receive will come from natural foods—no pills, no far-out dishes—simply the foods you already like and enjoy.

Why the emphasis on iron from natural food and no use of artificial supplements?

You don't want too much iron. It can be harmful—or even fatal. The human body has developed no quick, efficient way to get rid of large amounts, so quantities ever increase if doses way above the RDA are constantly taken; and excessive amounts of iron over a long period of time cause liver and pancreas damage, and adversely affect the heart. This can be seen in a primitive tribe of the Bantu group in South Africa. They use iron kettles to cook their food and brew their beer, and so much iron from the kettles gets into their systems (more than 250 mg per day, or over ten times the RDA) that they display the symptoms of iron poisoning.

Persons in the United States who take in too much iron from iron supplements encounter the same hazard—and another. A heavy dose of iron all at once can poison you immediately. Children who find their mother's iron tablets and empty the bottle court serious trouble—deaths have been reported.

So get your iron from natural foods. That way, you'll run no risk, for yourself, or for others.

FOODS FOR IRON

Richest in iron are meats and organs. Three ounces of lean hamburger contain 3 mg of iron, as do three ounces of steak. The same amount of liver yields 5 mg of iron. Liver, of course, is a storehouse of this mineral.

Some shellfish are high in iron. Three ounces of clam meat provide over 5 mg of iron. And a cup of oysters contains a whopping 13.6 mg!

Dark-green vegetables, such as spinach and peas, are good sources of iron. Another is dried fruits. Many cereals are now enriched with iron. A glance through the Appendix will reveal other foods that offer this mineral.

Peculiarly, milk, nature's nearly perfect food and the one in which mothers first transmit nutrients to their young, is badly lacking in iron. There is less than a milligram of iron in every two quarts of milk.

One source which supplied us with a little iron in the past has now been lost to advances in taste and technology. Iron cookware, with which the Bantu are all too familiar, at one time furnished small amounts of iron to the foods cooked in them and in turn to us. Iron for pots, of course, has given way to aluminum and Teflon. Practically no iron comes from the use of stainless steel ware.

6

CALCIUM: DEFICIENCY OF CRUMBLING BONES

FROM CHEMISTRY TO NUTRITION

The element calcium was discovered in 1808 by the brilliant English chemist Sir Humphry Davy. Though perhaps a genius, Davy, who also isolated potassium, sodium, magnesium, and boron, had the habit of identifying chemicals by tasting them—a mental if not dietary indiscretion—and managed to die young.

A French scientist, Chossat, fared better and demonstrated with experiments on pigeons that animals have a nutritional need for calcium. But it remained to twentieth-century researchers to prove that humans, too, required this mineral in their diets.

Calcium is the fifth most abundant element in the earth's crust, and in its pure form is a relatively soft, white metal; however, it is never found in its free state in nature, but generally as a part of salts, a class of chemical compounds often composed of metals, oxygen, and other substances in a certain molecular arrangement, usually crystalline in type. Calcium sulfate is a common salt present in the ground in gypsum. Another calcium salt, calcium phosphate, constitutes the principal structural material in animals: bones and teeth, the shell of eggs, sea shells—and in humans, bones and teeth.

FUNCTIONS OF CALCIUM

Most calcium in the human body, 99 percent, goes to make up bones and teeth, but a little is found dispersed throughout the blood and soft tissues, where it performs numerous odd tasks.

Our bones, of course, hold us up. They are analogous to the steel girders in a skyscraper. Just as these girders form a skeleton to shape and safeguard the interior, so our bones make a skeleton that shapes us and protects our vital organs—the skull shields the brain, the rib cage surrounds the heart and lungs.

But bones are more marvelous than steel girders. Not only do they give us shape and protection, they provide firm attachment for muscles, become larger as we grow, and mend themselves if broken. Bones also act as reservoirs for calcium in the blood stream—to keep the supply of this precious nutrient constant. If we ingest more calcium than we need, the excess is stored in the bones; if we take in too little, calcium in the bones finds its way into the circulatory system. So strong bones are mandatory to good health—and adequate intake of calcium is imperative for strong bones.

The same is true of teeth. Teeth cut and grind food and give shape to the jaw; and calcium is the chief component of tooth enamel, the white outer layer of the teeth, which is the hardest tissue in the human body.

But calcium is more than just a structural element.

It must be present in the blood for clotting to take place. In fact, hospitals often give patients injections of calcium salt before an operation to promote needed later coagulation.

Calcium is vital to body chemistry in other ways: for the rhythmic beating of the heart, contraction of muscles, transmission of nerve impulses, and many chemical reactions involving hormones and enzymes.

DWARFED, BRITTLE, AND BROKEN

What happens when the body does not get enough calcium?

Results vary with different age groups—but children suffer most.

Without dietary calcium, their growth is stunted and their bones weaken, with leg bones bowing outward, bending because of the weight of the body. A shrunken and deformed rib cage may be evident, as might a too-narrow jaw, which crowds the teeth. Female children face an added complication: a pelvis developing too narrow for easy childbirth. These are the symptoms of the disease called rickets.

Childhood also demands calcium for the strong, healthy teeth of future years, for the permanent teeth begin forming even before birth; and once the permanent teeth are fully evolved, they are little affected by calcium intake of later life. And the health of the baby teeth should not be passed over, since poor baby teeth may hinder the spacing and orientation of the permanent teeth.

Bad teeth, of course, inhibit the cutting and grinding of food, so eating must often be restricted to whatever foods the teeth can handle, which in turn may lead to an imbalanced diet, causing other deficiencies—a snowballing effect. Old folks with poor teeth commonly incur this type of imbalance and require attention from their physicians.

And without sufficient calcium, older people face more problems. If calcium intake in adults drops too low to cover the body's needs, then this mineral will be taken out of the bones to supply the blood and softer tissues, where it is indispensable to many processes. When this leaching occurs, the bones become weak and brittle, and much more vulnerable to breaking.

A certain amount of decalcification of the bones takes place as old age creeps up, in any case. But sometimes the condition becomes severe, and when this happens, its victims are said to have osteoporosis, a state characterized by fragile bones. Inadequate intake of calcium is thought to contribute to the severity and frequency of osteoporosis.

The chief sufferers of osteoporosis, as is true of most deficiency-related maladies in this country, are women. It is estimated that as many as 14 million women in the United States have this disease. Undoubtedly, this is why so many grandmothers and older aunts seem to be the ones who break their hips. When the aging ones fall, they usually sit down hard, putting great pressure on already weakened bones, fracturing them.

Osteoporosis is one of the reasons that nutritionists advocate a steady supply of calcium throughout middle age; they believe it will prevent excessive calcium erosion of bones in later years.

Other reasons: at least one study has shown that adequate amounts of calcium help keep cholesterol levels down; and a second study indicates that calcium may aid in the absorption of vitamin B-12, another essential nutrient.

CALCIUM, AMERICANS, AND DIETING

The calcium deficiency situation in the United States is almost as grave as that of the shortfall of dietary iron.

Females aged nine to thirty-four years range 21 to 29 percent below the RDA for calcium; and women thirty-five years of age and older average 30 percent or more below the RDA. Men fare a little better: males aged nine to seventeen are less than 10 percent below the RDA, as are men aged thirty-five to fifty-four; men over fifty-five years tend to fall 11 to 20 percent below the RDA. One group of males seems to be getting enough calcium: the eighteen-to-thirty-four-year-olds.

But on the whole, calcium deficiency is a serious problem. And persons going on reducing diets, already close to the edge of calcium deficiency, may drift over the boundary into real trouble, chancing the conditions we've discussed. This is especially true if they pattern their eating habits on some exotic diet plan that's badly lacking in calcium, as many are.

But the diet plans in Chapters Fifteen and Sixteen do not share this fault.

They've been designed for weight loss without stinting on calcium, furnishing the user with at least 800 mg of calcium daily, which is the adult RDA for this mineral. If you let these sensible diet plans guide your eating, as you lose weight, lack of calcium will not interfere with your health—nor will it come back to haunt you in future years.

THE FOUNT OF CALCIUM

Milk is far and away the best source of calcium.

A single cup of milk contains nearly 300 mg—or over one-third the RDA. Drink three cups a day and you need not worry about calcium.

But many people do not drink milk.

Some simply do not like it. Others think milk is only for children. Yet without milk in the diet it's very difficult to get enough calcium; and the need for calcium continues throughout all of life, as we have seen.

A large number of people avoid milk because they believe that it's fattening. There is some truth in this—a cup of milk contains 160 calories. For this reason skim milk is often used in diet plans. Skim milk differs from whole milk only in that the fat has been removed—the nutrition remains in. Taking the fat out of milk brings the calorie count down to 90 calories per cup, less than the number of calories in a cup of orange juice.

A few people are allergic to milk. Others have an intolerance for lactose, the carbohydrate in milk. These unfortunate people should be under the care of their physicians to insure that their diets are adequate.

So, if you're not in the last category, and you haven't done so already, you might learn to appreciate the value of milk, for the calcium that it holds—and the many other nutrients.

Other foods high in calcium are milk products, such as yogurt, cheeses, and real ice cream. Also good are the green vegetables, like spinach and broccoli. Meat and grain products are low in calcium.

7

THIAMIN:
THE FIRST VITAMIN

THE SEARCH

The staple food of southeast Asia is rice.

In the nineteenth century modern methods of rice milling were introduced to this region, and following this great technological advancement there surged a new outbreak of a fearsome disease already well known to the populace.

Beriberi.

The name is Singhalese (the language of Ceylon) and means "weakness."

The malady is aptly labeled. In its early stages victims suffer from numbness of the legs, cramps, and difficulty in walking. Later the legs become paralyzed and wasted, making locomotion impossible. Death usually marks the finish of the course of the disease.

And it was death by the thousands in the nineteenth century.

In the first years of the 1890s a Dutch physician, Christian Eijkman, while working in a military hospital in Java, became intrigued with the disease. Noticing that chickens sometimes suffered symptoms similar to those of beriberi, he studied these fowl intently. He first thought their sickness to be induced by microbes, but after vain attempts to establish this, he realized that invasion by microorganisms was not the answer. He turned his attention next to the food they ate and discovered that chickens fed with polished rice (rice from which the hulls had been removed, the new process) were the only ones felled by the disease. Chickens that consumed polished rice *and* the hulls were not affected. From this observation Eijkman reasoned that the polished rice contained a toxin which produced the disease and that the hulls held an antitoxin that nullified the powers of the chemical in the rice.

His deduction was logical—and wrong. But Eijkman was pointing inquiry in the right direction.

It was another Dutch physician, Grigns, who in 1901 suggested that beriberi and its counterpart in chickens sprang not from a poison in the diet, but from a lack of a specific substance that prevented the dreadful symptoms. In other words, he said, beriberi was a disease of deficiency, the missing of a nutrient required by the body.

This hypothesis launched an intense hunt in food for the supposed substance—soon to be termed a vitamin.

Yet, twenty years of laborious scientific research passed before the isolation of the elusive material was at last achieved; in 1926, a white powder, smelling like yeast and tasting something like salted nuts, removed vitamins from the realm of the mysterious and gave scientists a solid grasp on the combating of deficiency diseases.

And for the first time in its 2000 years of recorded history, the cloak of enigma was stripped away from beriberi, revealing it as simply a result of the dietary lack of the white powder—thiamin.

Obtaining pure thiamin was not easy. In the end a ton of rice had to be reduced to yield a few grams of it. And more years of hard work had to be undergone before thiamin was synthesized in the laboratory—this feat accomplished in 1936.

Patent royalties from the synthesis of thiamin since that time have financed research into nutrition in the United States and elsewhere throughout the world.

FUNCTIONS OF THIAMIN

Some of this research has established thiamin's role in body chemistry. This nutrient is now known to play an essential part in the breaking down of carbohydrates for the release and use of energy in all cells of the body—one of the most basic processes to the maintenance of life. When thiamin is not present, pyruvic acid and other incompletely metabolized substances build up and impair or halt the work of the cells. So important is thiamin to unimpeded operation of the body that it is found in every single tissue in the human system.

Symptoms of the lack of thiamin develop quickly. In a research study, a group of volunteers was fed a diet that contained zero thiamin but which was adequate in all other nutrients. After a few weeks the subjects complained of fatigue, lassitude, and insomnia; they also lost their appetites and became depressed and irritable.

If the subjects had proceeded beyond this stage, the subjects would have been victimized by nausea and vomiting, their heartbeats would have slowed, and the muscles whinh push food through the intestines would have slackened, causing constipation. Quickly confusion and fear would have dominated their mental states. Continued deprivation of thiamin would have terminated in outright beriberi, which lays waste the nerves, resulting in paralysis of the legs, and eventually, heart failure.

A tragic end for want of a few white crystals.

ALCOHOLICS AND FADDISTS

Beriberi is still prevalent throughout Asia; but severe thiamin deficiency in the United States is rare. One group of people in the United States which is deficient in thiamin, however, are the chronic alcoholics. Since nearly all of their calorie intake comes in the form of alcohol, with alcohol containing practically no nutrients, their nutritional inadequacies are sometimes appalling—often going far beyond simple thiamin deficiency. Many alcoholics contract Wernicke's disease, which produces eye problems, and Korsakoff's syndrome, in which confusion and forgetfulness govern the behavior of the victim. The two ailments, seemingly related, if caught early enough, can be cured by the administration of thiamin.

Another group which suffers from thiamin deficiency is the food faddists. These people often center their diets around one or two foods which lack this important nutrient. Concentrate on a diet like this long enough, and one could join the ranks of the thousands of Asians who know beriberi first hand.

For the population of the United States as a whole, a government study conducted in 1965 showed that the average intake of thiamin fell below the RDA for women of all age groups. Boys twelve to fourteen years old scored under the RDA; men placed above.

Of course, dieting can affect the situation adversely.

But if you follow the diet plans in Chapters Fifteen and Sixteen, you'll be assured of receiving at least 1.0 mg of thiamin daily, the RDA for women, a more-than-adequate amount for safety.

Doses larger than this, according to scientific research, in no way promote additional measures of good health. By its presence thiamin does prevent paralysis of the legs; but great amounts of it will not develop powerful limbs capable of tremendous athletic accomplishment. Thiamin may also be said to prevent depression, because its absence creates it; but huge quantities do not provide any extra life to spirits or induce mood changes. The "more is better" theory just does not apply.

While large doses of thiamin greatly in excess of the RDA provide no benefit, neither do they appear to be harmful, in contrast to some other vitamins. The body is able to store only a small quantity of this nutrient, and because thiamin is water soluble, most of any extra amount is quickly excreted in the urine.

SOURCES OF THIAMIN

Grain products, such as cereal and bread, furnish the largest part of most people's daily intake of thiamin. Much of the natural thiamin has been refined out of these foods, but because of a thiamin-enrichment program begun during World War II, synthetic thiamin has been added back in to many items, and performs as a reliable substitute—because it is thiamin.

Meat (especially pork), legumes, nuts, milk products, fruits, and vegetables remain good sources of natural thiamin. A cup of orange juice provides 0.22 mg of thiamin—or about 22 percent of the RDA for women. The best source of thiamin, however, is a substance which the average person seldom eats: yeast! It's loaded with it.

When preparing foods with thiamin, beware of dry heating processes, such as baking. This method of preparation can cause considerable destruction of the nutrient. On the other hand, moist cooking affects it very little—unless cooking time is unusually prolonged. But use water sparingly, since significant amounts of the vitamin can be lost to it.

Baking soda, also the enemy of other nutrients, completely destroys thiamin and should be used sparingly in cooking.

8

NIACIN:
PLUCKED FROM CONFUSION

FITTING THE PIECES

Nutritional scientists were puzzled.

Over the years in their search for the pellagra-preventing (p-p) factor in food, they were obtaining confusing results.

The problem had its origins in 1867.

In that year a German chemist, Huber, manufactured a substance he called nicotinic acid from nicotine, the deadly poison found in tobacco plants. But at that time any possible connection of the new chemical to nutrition went unguessed, and for a long while nicotinic acid remained just another white powder in flasks cluttering laboratory shelves.

Yet by 1912 scientists were beginning to find nicotinic acid and a related compound named nicotinamide (the two substances together called niacin in America) in foods, and shortly thereafter, in tissues of the human body.

Still, any significance of niacin to nutrition or deficiency disease was missed. In fact, some scientists, unconcerned with pellagra, dismissed the relevancy of niacin to deficiency disease because in their experiments niacin did not cure beriberi!

Meanwhile, Goldberger was working on pellagra.

At first he suspected that pellagra stemmed from a dietary deficiency of an amino acid, a chemical link in the chain that forms protein molecules. But then his research led him to believe that an unknown dietary factor was involved, probably a yet-to-be-discovered vitamin. He proved that this p-p factor was present in yeast after thiamin was destroyed. But he was not able to uncover its identity. He did not connect niacin with the problem.

At the same time, research by others appeared to indicate that it was indeed an amino acid, tryptophan, that was the culprit in pellagra, as Goldberger had first thought. Milk diets, high in tryptophan, were given to pellagrans, curing them of the disease.

Now there were two solutions to the pellagra problem. Who, then, was right? The backers of tryptophan? Or Goldberger, who believed the cause to be the lack of a vitamin?

Further studies seemed to cloud the picture.

Niacin, now coming under scrutiny at last, when fed to dogs, rid them of blacktongue, the pellagra of the canine species. And niacin was proved to be present in yeast after thiamin destruction (as Goldberger had determined the unknown p-p factor to be), both circumstances lending support to Goldberger's theory of vitamin involvement. But when a corn-centered diet was analyzed, the diet of many pellagrans, researchers, who believed there would be little niacin, were startled to discover that corn is much higher in niacin than milk, the curer of pellagra in humans—a paradox, if the lack of niacin was indeed the cause of this malady.

What was the answer?

Scientists finally resolved the issue after World War II when they discovered that tryptophan, the amino acid in milk, is a precursor of the vitamin niacin.

In the human body, a chemical process turns tryptophan into niacin, much as carotene becomes vitamin A. This is the reason for the confusion in the search for the p-p factor among the various chemicals, foods, and diets. Milk is low in actual niacin, the pellagra-related nutrient; but milk contains eight times the equivalent amount of niacin in the form of tryptophan—which explains why milk is effective in the treatment of pellagra, whereas corn, which does contain some niacin (but not enough) is not.

But it is niacin which proved to be the much-sought-after pellagra-preventing factor. In the end, Goldberger was vindicated.

NIACIN AND DIETING

Niacin plays a complex role in body chemistry, and like thiamin, it is involved with the metabolism of carbohydrates in cells. Without niacin, cell chemistry is wrecked; and it is this impaired functioning that leads to the condition known as pellagra.

Is the diet of the average American adequate in niacin?

The answer in general is yes; but on occasion niacin deficiency does appear in people with certain medical problems, such as diabetes, tuberculosis, and gastrointestinal disorders. It can also be seen in people who have faulty diets: the poor, the chronic alcoholics, and our old friends the food faddists.

Dieting for weight reduction, as it does for many nutrients, also raises a question of sufficient amounts. Experimenting with foods and diet plans may disturb niacin ingestion. However, the diet plans in Chapters Fifteen and Sixteen provide at least 13 mg of niacin daily, which is the RDA for adult women; and the tryptophan present in the menus supplies additional quantities, increasing the safety factor.

The niacin in the diet plans comes from natural foods; and because of this, you can be assured that although you'll receive enough of it for good health, you'll not get too much, which can cause problems. Extra heavy doses of niacin produce flushing of the face, dizziness, a feeling of intense heat and itching, nausea, vomiting, and diarrhea. Continued overdosage eventually leads to liver disturbances.

Since the lack of niacin can cause mental breakdown, massive doses of it have been tried in cases of schizophrenia—but with no effect as a remedy. If the mental disorder does not derive from the deficiency of niacin, then this nutrient will not function as a cure.

Large amounts of niacin have also been tested as a palliative for coronary disease; but scientists can find no evidence that niacin influences mortality rates among heart-attack victims.

Researchers experimenting with volunteers have found that four grams of nicotinic acid per day, over 300 times the recommended amount, can reduce blood cholesterol levels by about 11 percent. But the side effects are a heavy price to pay for this reduction, especially when other methods of lowering cholesterol exist that are much safer.

SOURCES OF NIACIN

Foods with plentiful amounts of niacin or tryptophan are meats, eggs, and milk. Poultry is an especially excellent source. Whole or enriched grains are also good, as is yeast, the favorite hiding spot of thiamin. Of the two forms of niacin, nicotinic acid comes from plants, and nicotinamide from animals.

Niacin is one of the most indestructable of vitamins. It resists heat, light, and oxidation. But since niacin is water-soluble, use as little water as possible when you cook foods containing it—to conserve as much as possible of this valuable nutrient.

9

RIBOFLAVIN:
THE LUMINOUS VITAMIN

A PECULIAR CHARACTERISTIC

Shortly after World War I scientists discovered the need for another vitamin beyond that of thiamin.

They found that when they heated yeast for several hours, the vitamin which prevented beriberi was destroyed, but a second factor which promoted growth in rats remained. In reality several nutrients, the first one of the new group to be studied, was given the name of Vitamin B2 by British researchers and vitamin G by Americans. In 1932 the name *riboflavin* was decided upon when more experiments determined the nutrient to be made up of *ribose* (a sugar) and *flavus* (a pigment).

Riboflavin in its pure form consists of crystals which are orange-yellow in color. They are odorless but taste bitter. The crystals are soluble in water, and once they dissolve, the solution becomes greenish-yellow. If you were to look closely at this solution, you would notice something interesting about it: it glows! Riboflavin has the property of fluorescence; that is, when light falls upon it, it seems to shine with a light of its own. This curious property of riboflavin is in no way connected with its function as a vitamin.

VARIETY OF DUTIES

Riboflavin performs several jobs in the human body. Like thiamin and niacin, it plays a significant part in cell respiration, in which hydrogen is "burned" with oxygen to make water, releasing energy required for life functions. For this reason, it is found in nearly every cell in the body. Riboflavin also aids in the production of red blood cells and is thought to be important in making retinal pigments, substances in the eyeball necessary for good vision. It also helps convert tryptophan to niacin—yet another instance of one vitamin assisting another.

Researchers guess that riboflavin plays other roles in maintaining good health; these contributions will be uncovered in the years to come as scientists slowly unravel the mysteries of nutrition and the human body.

DEFICIENCY

Riboflavin deficiency has devastating results in animals: growth failure, sudden collapse, and death. But in man the effects are less drastic.

The first scientific study of riboflavin deficiency in humans was conducted in 1939. Eighteen healthy women were fed a diet lacking riboflavin but sufficient in all the other nutrients. The women developed fissures in the angles of the mouth, lesions on the lips, and greasy skin around the nose. The experiment was halted; and when the women were fed riboflavin, all adverse conditions disappeared, as is usually the case with mild vitamin deficiencies and subsequent ingestion of the missing nutrient.

Severe riboflavin deficiency, as is sometimes seen in underdeveloped nations, leads to pronounced medical problems. One of the first symptoms is burning of the eyes. Progressively, the tongue becomes magenta in color (as opposed to the bright red of pellagra), the skin on the face takes on a greasy appearance, and after a time anemia arises. Dermatitis of the scrotum may also occur in men.

The most calamitous effect, however, is on the eyes. Vision becomes clouded; and occasionally the cornea turns completely opaque, blinding the victim.

In contrast to animals, in humans there are no known cases of death from riboflavin deficiency. This may be due to the fact that bacteria which live in our intestines produce some riboflavin, which we absorb—perhaps enough to keep us alive. In return for the riboflavin, the bacteria feed on a little of the food that passes through the intestinal tract. This is a fair exchange, the partnership between man and microbe benefiting both.

An aside—I once received in the mail a booklet that advertised vitamins, laxatives, and other such things. Part of the literature described in vivid terms a drug that would kill the millions of bacteria that live in our intestines. Be bacteria-free, was the pitch. But what the advertisement did not say, of course, was that these microorganisms in no way harm the body, but actually promote good health, and should remain unmolested!

In fact, bacteria help with the supply of riboflavin in another way—besides human intestinal production—by allowing cows to digest grass, which in turn becomes milk loaded with riboflavin, a major source of this nutrient for humans.

At one time riboflavin deficiency was quite common in the southern part of the United States where milk consumption was low; but today the situation has changed for the better, thanks in large measure to general improvement in eating habits, and also to the cereal-enrichment program, which was begun in 1941.

However, at present there is a disturbing trend toward decreased intake of riboflavin among women. This backsliding may be attributed to the drop in milk consumption affecting all of us in recent years, and to the fact that women are more weight-conscious than men. When thoughts of weight control and dieting strike, women tend to eat what they think of as "less fattening" foods, often at the expense of riboflavin and their nutritional health.

But as a dieter, man or woman, you will not have to worry about this problem. By following the diet plans in Chapters Fifteen and Sixteen, not only will you lose weight, you'll also get plenty of riboflavin, at least 1.5 mg daily, more than the RDA for adult women—and you'll receive all the other nutrients you need to reduce and stay healthy.

10

VITAMIN E:
THE VITAMIN PROTECTOR

A WONDER DRUG?

As a substance with miraculous capabilities, probably more claims have been made for vitamin E in normal and heavy doses than for any other single nutrient. At one time or another, it has been said to be a curer of sexual impotence, multiple sclerosis, heart disease, and skin disorders; that it helps blood circulation and athletic ability; and that it slows the aging process.

Is any of this true?

Let's look at vitamin E, its properties, functions in the body, deficiency and overdosage problems, and dietary requirements, to see if there is any basis in fact for these oft-stated claims, and whether or not a reducing diet might deprive the body of vitamin E and its supposed extraordinary boosting powers to good health.

CHARACTERISTICS

Seven chemical compounds are found in nature that have vitamin E activity; and science has produced another several dozen synthetic compounds that also have vitamin E activity in the human body. Of these, the naturally occurring compound α- tocopherol is the most potent. Vitamin E, as we will call all of these substances, is a thick oil, pale yellow in color, soluble in fat but not in water.

Vitamin E has only one definitely known function in the human body. It is an antioxidant. That is, it prevents the deterioration of vital materials in the body by not allowing them to combine with oxygen—so that they do not spoil and lose their utility. Vitamin E soaks up oxygen, peroxides, and fragments of other molecules that are highly reactive and that can be extremely damaging to cells, thus protecting the functioning of the human system from the impairment and breakdown that these substances would otherwise cause. Vitamin E also keeps vitamin A from oxidizing, preserving the usefulness of this nutrient for the many body processes in which it must participate, a case of one vitamin helping another, not an unusual occurrence.

But if this is all that vitamin E does, then what about all those fabulous claims? The unfortunate truth is that they are distortions, which probably stem from a combination of the original vitamin E deficiency studies and a liberal coating of the "if a little is good, then more must be better" theory that seems to fascinate and guide so many people. For instance, the idea that vitamin E is a sex vitamin and can cure impotence undoubtedly originates from studies of rats that show vitamin E is necessary for reproduction. If vitamin E is needed for correct progression from conception to birth, it is argued, then massive doses of it must promote increased potency. Alas, this belief is fallacious. While vitamin E *is* necessary for the successful conclusion of the reproductive process, science can find no evidence that a large amount of this nutrient in any way improves the quality or quantity of sex life.

Misunderstanding of the studies of vitamin E and animals has misled the public about this vitamin and its relation to multiple sclerosis and heart disease. Deficiency of vitamin E in experimental animals can cause these maladies. However, multiple sclerosis in man does not, unfortunately, respond to vitamin E treatment; and scientists have uncovered no evidence that it is helpful in the fight against heart disease.

Similarly, there is no proof that vitamin E is a palliative for skin disorders.

On the other hand, any connection between vitamin E and

blood circulation remains ambiguous. Some studies seem to show that it is an aid to circulation, while others indicate that it is not. This area awaits more intensive research.

But as far as enhancing athletic ability with vitamin E, an extensive study has already produced concrete answers. In Britain, researchers divided schoolboys into two groups of 15 boys each, one group receiving vitamin E in tablet form and the other group receiving an identical-looking tablet that did not contain the nutrient. Neither group knew who was taking the vitamin E. The boys embarked on a swimming program and their physical fitness was monitored as they progressed. Over the weeks of the study fitness improved, as could be expected with any exercise program, but neither group outperformed the other, indicating that vitamin E had no effect on athletic ability.

Finally, what about aging and vitamin E? We know that red blood cells live a shorter period of time if deprived of vitamin E. But whether they or other human cells would live beyond their normal life spans in the body when supplied with extra amounts of vitamin E as yet remains to be determined. Research is currently being conducted into this area, and the results are awaited with great interest.

In the meantime, be wary of large amounts of vitamin E.

One scientist reports that he felt fatigue when he experimented with ingesting over 50 times the RDA of this nutrient daily. In a more controlled study, researchers found decreased levels of red blood cells in chickens fed massive doses of vitamin E, which looks suspiciously like a case of vitamin overdosage producing the same effects as the related deficiency, an outcome we know can happen.

VITAMIN E REQUIREMENTS AND DIETING

The RDA for vitamin E was set for the first time in 1968 and was established at 30 International Units (30 IU) per day for adult men and women. In the light of new studies the RDA was revised downward in 1974 to 12 IU for women and 15 IU for men.

Because of the plentiful supply of vitamin E in the American diet, vitamin E deficiency is exceedingly rare in the United States.

When it does make its appearance, the only observable symptom of deficiency is a slight decrease in the life span of red blood cells in the circulatory system—vitamin E no longer protecting them from destructive oxidation. Presumably, this condition would eventually lead to anemia. The pervasiveness of vitamin E in food, however, and the length of time it takes to deplete stores of it in the liver—2.5 years—makes this development unlikely.

Good sources of vitamin E include salad oils, margarine, and green leafy vegetables. Liver also ranks high in this nutrient. Even potato chips contain significant amounts of vitamin E. The best natural source is wheat germ oil.

Vitamin E is resistant to heat, and since it does not dissolve in water, little of it is lost in cooking or in the pasteurization of milk. It can, however, be processed out of food—for example, when whole wheat is turned into white bread. But this loss is offset by the fact that many other foods are enriched with vitamin E because of its antioxidant property, which keeps foods from becoming rancid.

Since vitamin E acts as a preservative and is not in any way a wonder drug, you do not relinquish any miraculous benefits you might obtain from this vitamin by decreasing your intake of food when dieting. Neither do you have to risk supplementation of your diet with pills or capsules.

Of course, a certain amount of vitamin E is necessary for good health. But it is not a nutrient to worry about as you diet. The reducing plans in Chapters Fifteen and Sixteen, well-balanced, will provide adequate amounts.

11

THE REMAINING REGULATORS: IODINE, VITAMIN D, AND OTHERS

IODINE

Iodine is a blue-gray solid that produces a dense violet vapor when heated; and when put into alcohol mixed with water, it makes the purple-colored solution of tincture of iodine, the well-known antiseptic used for treating cuts.

Iodine has another role. It is requisite in microscopic amounts for proper functioning of the human body and is the most important ingredient of thyroid hormones, the substances which control basal metabolic rate, the idling speed of the body which we will discuss in Chapter Thirteen.

When iodine is not present in the human system, the thyroid gland, which is located just under the Adam's apple in the throat, entarges in an effort to compensate for the lack of this mineral, creating the condition called *goiter*, a huge swelling in the front of the neck.

Goiter is one of the oldest diseases depicted by mankind. Chinese records of 3000 B.C. describe goiter, and paintings of goitrous persons can be found in European art throughout the ages.

But goiter is not only a malady of the past—today 200 million people of the earth's population are afflicted with iodine deficiency and the resulting unsightly growth of the thyroid gland.

Although extensive, incidence of goiter is not evenly distributed over the globe. Availability and ingestion of foods containing iodine govern its prevalence. Because iodine is a component of salts in sea water that become a part of seafood, and because salt particles in sea spray can be wafted for miles inland to crops that absorb the minerals in them, goiter is usually absent from coastal areas. Conversely, mountainous regions and lands far from the sea generally experience a much higher occurrence of goiter—with Switzerland having the highest rate of all nations. In countries like this, where goiter is endemic over many generations, infants are often born with too little thyroid hormone and start life as victims of *cretinism*, a condition caused by the lack of thyroid hormone and characterized by deformity, dwarfism, and imbecility. (The word *cretin* comes from a French dialect and means "Christian," the term being used as an expression of pity.) These unfortunate creatures usually do not live beyond early adulthood.

Happily, cretinism is not endemic in the United States—but goiter is not unknown. A national survey conducted a few years ago reveals that one person in every twenty in this country has an enlarged thyroid gland—because of iodine deficiency. As usual, women are the hardest hit, the condition showing up in five times as many females as males. The problem is largely due to the varying iodine content of foods.

And iodine deficiency may be aggravated by dieting—when food selection is modified in some fashion. But any trouble can be avoided, however, by eating foods rich in natural iodine (which may be difficult to do because of location) or by the use of iodized salt (salt in which an occasional chlorine atom has been replaced by an atom of iodine—not changing taste or price) for seasoning purposes.

The taking of concentrated iodine supplements, such as in the form of seaweed tablets and the like, is definitely not recommended, since amounts only 25 times the RDA have proven toxic to the human system.

If you don't already employ it on your table, iodized salt is an addition you might consider making to the diet plans outlined in Chapters Fifteen and Sixteen. (Be sure the label says "iodized." Unlike the salt sold in Canada and other countries, not all salt sold in the United States is iodized.)

VITAMIN D

Rickets, the bone disease we talked about in the chapter on calcium, like goiter, has plagued man across time and national boundaries. The ancient Greeks described it in much the same terms that nutritionists and doctors use today in modern medical journals. And the ailment was so common among English children in the last century that it was dubbed the "English disease."

As we know, rickets can be caused by the lack of dietary calcium, but it's far more likely to be induced by a dearth of vitamin D, for this nutrient is the agent that makes possible the removal of calcium from food and its deposition on the bones—a process requisite for strength and structural integrity. This is also true for calcium in teeth—vitamin D is a must.

The existence of vitamin D was unmasked in the 1920s when researchers close on the trail of the unknown growth-promoting nutrients discovered that cod-liver oil in which all the vitamin A had been destroyed still contained a substance that experiments proved both prevented and cured rickets. Some years later the nutrient was given the name vitamin D, assuming its place in line alphabetically behind vitamin C.

A nutrient resistant to breakdown, vitamin D in pure form consists of colorless crystals that dissolve in fats and oils but not in water.

Researchers in their probings uncovered an interesting aspect of this new nutrient: there are few good natural food sources of it. How then does man obtain enough vitamin D?

From sunshine!

Scientists found that cholesterol (an alcohol found in animal fats) located in the cells just beneath the surface of the skin changes into vitamin D when "tickled" with a little ultraviolet light, the same radiation from the sun that excites the pigment-producing cells into giving us a tan.

Some animals appear also to utilize sunshine as a source of vitamin D. Apparently when a dog licks his coat or a bird preens his feathers, they are not doing it for grooming purposes only. On the hair and feathers is an oil that contains a substance which turns into vitamin D when sunlight strikes it. As the animal grooms, the vitamin passes into his system.

In general, man does not need much vitamin D. The Food and Nutrition Board has set the adult RDA at 400 IU (International Units—a very small measure) daily. Some vitamin D can be gotten by eating fish, such as salmon, herring, sardines, and tuna, and cod-liver oil; it can also be obtained by drinking milk fortified with vitamin D.

But the worry is not getting enough vitamin D—the hazard is receiving too much. An overdose of only twenty times the RDA can cause vomiting, diarrhea, and kidney damage. Higher doses will actually remove calcium from the bones and clog blood vessels with it. Pregnant women ingesting several thousand times the RDA daily through supplements will give birth to mentally retarded children.

So, as you diet, don't take vitamin D pills; instead drink skim milk fortified with vitamin D—this is a good way to receive the right amount of this nutrient. Or for a time each day, not overdoing it, go outside and enjoy the sunshine!

FOLACIN

Folacin is a name given to several substances that have similar vitamin activity. One of them, folic acid, was first isolated in 1943 and manufactured in the laboratory in 1946. A yellow powder, folic acid is soluble in water.

Folacin in humans is necessary for the synthesis of nucleic acids (materials of genetic importance in the cells) and amino acids, the basic components of protein.

Lacking folacin, man develops a particular type of anemia called *macrocytic anemia,* a condition in which young red blood cells fail to mature, resulting in a lowered red-blood-cell count. As is usually the case with a deficiency disease and the corresponding missing nutrient, this form of anemia can be cured by the administration of folacin. Folacin, however, is not useful in fighting anemias arising from other causes. For instance, in iron-deficiency anemia, though the red-blood-cell count is low, the iron necessary for the formation of hemoglobin just is not present, and no amount of folacin will help.

More overt symptoms of folacin-associated anemia are a smooth red tongue and gastrointestinal disturbances.

Unlike dogs, rats, and rabbits, who have a set of bacteria in their intestines to synthesize it, human beings must get all of their folacin from the foods they eat. Consequently, an unbalanced diet can induce a folacin deficiency. This is especially true for pregnant women and lactating women, whose need for folacin is increased.

The Food and Nutrition Board has set the RDA for folacin at 400 micrograms (one microgram, abbreviated μg, equal to one one-millionth of a gram) daily for adults.

The best sources of folacin are green, leafy vegetables, liver, and yeast. But eating a balanced diet will supply enough of this nutrient.

VITAMIN K

Vitamin K is one of the four fat-soluble vitamins (A, D, E, and K). Yellow in color, vitamin K was first isolated in 1939, four years after the need for it was discovered.

To name this nutrient, the letter *k* was taken from the German word *Koagulation*, equivalent to the English word *coagulation*, chosen because vitamin K is an aid to the blood-clotting process.

Vitamin K deficiency delays or prevents blood clotting; and if this nutrient is not present, death from external or internal bleeding can result.

Vitamin K deficiency in man is rare, since bacteria in the intestine manufacture it. However, deficiency can be brought about by the killing of these bacteria, as with antibiotics, or by the hindrance of vitamin K absorption from the intestines to the bloodstream, an effect of certain medical conditions.

A good food source of vitamin K is the green, leafy vegetables, like spinach and lettuce. Liver and eggs also contain vitamin K.

Because of little knowledge about the contribution of vitamin K by intestinal bacteria to human nutrition, the RDA for this vitamin has yet to be fixed.

CHOLINE

Choline, a white, sirupy liquid soluble in water, was discovered to have vitamin activity when researchers demonstrated that its presence was necessary to prevent the accumulation of fat in the livers of experimental animals. Without choline, fatty deposits increase in the livers of rats, dogs, cats, pigs, and rabbits.

Choline deficiency in man, however, has never been seen; thus, no RDA has been set for this nutrient.

Food sources rich in choline include eggs, meat, whole grains, and legumes.

VITAMIN B-6

Vitamin B-6 is the name given to three naturally occurring compounds which have the same vitamin function. All three are white powders, soluble in water.

Vitamin B-6 is known to be important in amino-acid metabolism and is a requirement for the conversion of tryptophan to niacin.

Lack of vitamin B-6 in adults can cause dermatitis around the eyes and mouth, and a smooth, red tongue. Prolonged deficiency can bring on dizziness, confusion, nausea, vomiting, anemia, and convulsions.

Vitamin B-6 can be destroyed by heat; and it is this fact that led to the discovery of the need for vitamin B-6 in human nutrition. It happened in 1951 when signs of deficiency developed in infants fed a commercial baby food which had been sterilized by high heat, and investigators pinpointed the cause. (Today, care in baby-food preparation now prevents destruction of vitamin B-6).

The RDA of vitamin B-6 for adults in 2 mg daily.

Foods high in this nutrient are meats, liver, and yeast. Other sources are beans and whole grains.

VITAMIN B-12

A group of compounds called corrinoids, composed of red, water-soluble crystals, carry the name of *vitamin B-12*.

First isolated in 1948, vitamin B-12 has yet to be synthesized in the laboratory, since the molecules of this nutrient are large and complex. However, amounts can easily be derived from bacteria and fungi, which are the sole producers of vitamin B-12, grown in large vats.

An inadequate supply of vitamin B-12 to the human system can cause back pains, a sore tongue, physical weakness, and mental disorders. More importantly, however, it can bring on the associated deficiency disease, *pernicious anemia*, a condition characterized by reduced blood-cell count and degeneration of the spinal column, which, if left untreated, always proves fatal.

Deficiency can be incurred by lack of vitamin B-12 in the diet, or by faulty absorption of it from the intestinal tract. If the latter is the case, then the ailment is treated by injection of the nutrient directly into the blood stream.

Vitamin B-12 finds its way from bacteria and fungi into meats, seafood, eggs, and milk. Because higher plants cannot manufacture it, only negligible amounts are found in them. Hence, anyone on a vegetarian diet should include some eggs, milk, or their products, in his regimen.

The RDA for vitamin B-12 is set at 3.0 μg for adults.

PANTOTHENIC ACID

A water-soluble vitamin, pantothenic acid plays a role in breaking down foodstuffs for energy, as well as having other functions in the body.

This vitamin is found in every living cell, and under normal circumstances there is little likelihood of developing a deficiency disease from the lack of it. Symptoms can be produced when volunteers take a special drug that inhibits the action of the vitamin; when this occurs, the subjects note fatigue, nausea, and muscle cramps.

Foods rich in pantothenic acid are yeast, liver, eggs, and whole grains. Intestinal bacteria are believed to produce this nutrient in man.

An RDA for pantothenic acid has yet to be established.

BIOTIN

Biotin is a white, water-soluble vitamin which in man is produced by intestinal bacteria, thus eliminating the necessity of obtaining it from food sources and making deficiency rare.

Biotin deficiency can be induced by killing the biotin-creating bacteria with certain drugs, or by the eating of a great deal of raw egg white. Raw egg white contains a protein called avidin; and avidin combines with biotin in the intestines to form a compound that cannot be absorbed. Cooking the egg white destroys the action of avidin, however.

The infrequent deficiency of biotin results in listlessness, depression, and mild anemia.

An RDA for biotin has not been set.

SODIUM AND CHLORINE

The minerals sodium and chlorine are necessary in the body to maintain the proper balance between acidity and alkalinity. (We operate best in a slightly alkaline condition.)

They have other uses as well.

Sodium plays a part in the functioning of nerves and in regulating the amount of water held by the body; and chlorine is a major component of the digestive acid in the stomach, and also helps to kill alien microbes that enter the system with food.

Sodium and chlorine depletion can cause mental confusion and muscle cramps. Severe impoverishment will bring on coma and death.

Providentially, this last situation is unlikely, for sodium and chlorine are conveniently found together as common table salt (sodium chloride), which we sprinkle liberally on our food. In fact, the danger is not getting too little, but too much—because of our overuse of salt. Heavy sodium intake has been linked to high blood pressure. In places where salt ingestion is large, like Japan, high blood pressure is extensive.

In general, it's wise for most people to reduce their intake of salt. (The salt you do use should be iodized.)

PHOSPHORUS

Phosphorus, a nonmetallic element that glows in the dark, in conjunction with calcium gives bones and teeth their strength. It also plays other roles in body chemistry, such as in helping the blood to remain in proper acid-base balance, in cell division, and in reproductive processes.

Phosphorus deficiency can lead to weakness and bone pain. However, phorphorus deficiency is exceedingly rare, since this mineral is found in many foods. It will occasionally surface in a person who uses antacids over a long period of time; antacids render phosphorus unabsorbable.

MORE MINERALS

A number of other elements are important to body functioning. Magnesium is required for the release of energy in the cells and for the maintenance of the integrity of RNA and DNA, long chains of molecules involved in the transmission of hereditary characteristics. Another metal, copper, contributes to the prevention of anemia. Potassium is needed for the correct firing of nerve impulses. And fluorine helps to preserve the teeth.

These are not the only functions in which these elements participate. Nor have we discussed all the regulatory substances the body demands for good health. Dozens of others, in tiny amounts, have some part to play in the body's life processes. However, their nutritional properties have yet to be fully explored and their abundance in food measured. But by eating a well-balanced diet of natural foods, such as presented by the plans in Chapters Fifteen and Sixteen, you will be sure to get them.

12

THE ENERGY NUTRIENTS AND FIBER: CARBOHYDRATES, FAT, PROTEIN, AND CELLULOSE

A REVIEW AND MORE

Any substance found in foods that contributes to the operation of the body is called a *nutrient*. Over forty of them are known. Nutrients can be catalogued in several ways; but generally they might be divided into two classes: those which aid in the regulation of chemical processes, the vitamins and to a certain extent the minerals; and those which provide energy so that all the functions of the body may be carried out—carbohydrates, fat, and protein.

In addition to the two classes of nutrients, there exists in food a material which is usually not thought of as a nutrient but which just the same seems to be a part of the diet necessary for good health: fiber.

Most foods contain a number of nutrients and some fiber: but by far the most abundant substances in food are the energy nutrients: carbohydrates, fat, and protein.

We've mentioned them in passing, but now it's time we looked at them in more detail, for they have other duties to perform in the body besides supplying energy—functions that can be affected by dieting. (Energy and obesity will be discussed in Part II.)

And, as we probe the energy nutrients, we'll also say a few words about fiber.

CARBOHYDRATES

Carbohydrates are compounds formed from carbon, hydrogen, and oxygen atoms that we know more familiarly as sugars, starches, and cellulose—the last two in reality substances made from the complex combination of sugar molecules.

The simple sugars include glucose, fructose, and galactose. Glucose is the sugar carried by the blood stream that supplies energy to the cells. Hospital patients often receive glucose transfusions to bolster their energy resources. Fructose is the sugar found in fruits, and, along with glucose, it also is present in honey. Galactose occurs in the body, an important component of tissue.

When two simple sugars combine, they form what is known as a double sugar, or a disaccharide. Sucrose, the familiar sugar we buy at the supermarket (usually made from sugar cane) is a disaccharide, a combination of fructose and galactose. Another disaccharide is lactose, the sugar in milk; lactose is composed of glucose and galactose.

Starch consists of three or four hundred glucose molecules linked together in a long chain. Easily digested, starch is the chief source of energy in foods derived from plants.

Cellulose is another carbohydrate formed from long chains of glucose; but in contrast to starch, cellulose, a fiber, is not digestible in the human system. Cellulose also comes from plants—where it gives them structural strength.

Carbohydrates are often thought of as dietary villains, believed to be fattening by many people and pictured as poisonous to the body by others. This is definitely *not* the case. Carbohydrates are indispensable parts of the human diet. Even indigestible cellulose has its use, as we shall see.

Are carbohydrates automatically fattening?

For human beings, foods composed largely of carbohydrates are the cheapest and most plentiful sources of energy on earth. Much of the world's poor eat carbohydrate foods almost exclusively; they cannot afford fat or protein. Their diet is very high in carbohydrates, but they are not fat. As we shall see, it is the number of calories that count in weight loss and gain, and not the source of the energy. The world's poor are skin and bones despite their diet of carbohydrates.

Moreover, carbohydrates are not poisonous to the system. In fact, the body stores a carbohydrate called glycogen in the liver, where it is used to detoxicate real poisons that are accidentally swallowed—certainly a valuable service. Glycogen also acts as an emergency source of energy supply.

Dietary carbohydrates have other functions. Whenever caloric expenditure exceeds caloric intake, the body brings fat out of storage from the fatty tissues and metabolizes it to make up the energy deficit. And dietary carbohydrate must be on hand to help oxidize the fat. The process breaks down without it. If carbohydrates are missing from the diet, and this state is actually aimed at and central to some reducing plans, then the fat molecules will be incompletely metabolized and will remain a class of chemical called *ketones*.

Having too many ketones in the body results in a condition known as *ketosis*. And that's bad. Perhaps the least serious consequence of ketosis is foul breath. Ketones are exhaled from the lungs, giving the breath the smell of acetone (the odor of nail polish and certain glues used in model airplane construction). Other effects of ketosis are more grave. Ketones may cause the heart to beat irregularly, and for overweight people whose hearts are already taxed beyond normal limits this can be dangerous. Also, ketones irritate the kidneys, an unwelcome and potentially serious response for people with kidney disease. And ketosis aggravates symptoms of gout, ills which many gout sufferers already find unbearable. In pregnant women, ketosis can cause brain damage to unborn infants.

All in all, ketosis is a state to be avoided.

Other unpleasant side effects accompany a low-carbohydrate diet. A person on such a regimen generally feels weak and fatigued. He may become nauseous and sometimes fall victim to fainting. And his bowel movements will become labored and less regular—from the lack of fiber in his diet.

Fiber is an indigestible material (mostly cellulose) which adds bulk to the diet but not energy; and fiber in the human diet comes almost exclusively from carbohydrate foods; grains, fruits, and vegetables (especially the green, leafy kind).

By absorbing water, fiber makes the stools in the digestive tract large and soft; as a result, the stools move rapidly through the intestines, pushed easily along by the rings and bands of intestinal muscles.

Lacking fiber, stools grow small and hard; and when they do, the intestinal muscles, straining to thrust this type of stool ahead, become overdeveloped in some places and underdeveloped in others. Into the weakened muscular areas sometimes evolve tiny pouches, called *diverticula*, which can entrap small amounts of feces and become infected. When this happens, the victim is said to have *diverticulitis*, a malady usually accompanied by abdominal pain, and for which surgery is often the only alleviator.

But diverticulitis, as serious as it is, may only be a lesser hazard of the low fiber diet. Some scientists believe that the length of time stools spend in the intestine correlates closely with incidence of *cancer of the colon*—the longer the time, the greater the risk of cancer. From this, other researchers reason that since a high fiber content permits a much swifter passage of the stool, the incorporation into the diet of carbohydrate foods containing large amounts of fiber will decrease the chance of contracting this deadly disorder. (In regions throughout the world where the population subsists on a high-carbohydrate–high-fiber diet, cancer of the colon is rare.)

To prevent the above occurrences (the cancer question awaits definitive evidence), the Food and Nutrition Board recommends that Americans include carbohydrates in their diet. But because of the wide range of intake compatible with good health, the Board has not computed an RDA for this class of nutrient.

Foods of plant origin, such as cereals, bread, corn, and potatoes, are high in carbohydrates. Very little comes from animal sources, except for the lactose in milk.

FAT

Like the carbohydrates, *fat* is a chemical compound composed of carbon, hydrogen, and oxygen. But in fat these elements have a different arrangement and proportion, which gives fat a set of characteristics dissimilar to those of carbohydrates. There are several kinds of fat—but all are greasy to the touch and insoluble in water.

Most people think of fat as the scourge of the dietary-medical world. And in large amounts in the body it certainly can be such. A person who is overweight should shed any extra fat.

But we cannot dispense with all of it.

For like the other nutrients, fat has uses in the human system for which there is no substitute. In adipose (fatty) tissue fat resides as an energy store to be employed when food is scarce. Insulating the body against cold, fat also cushions vital organs. And fat is necessary in tissue structure, and for nerve-impulse transmission, the synthesis of hormones, and many other important functions. One of the building blocks of fat, an essential fatty acid called linoleic acid, by its presence in the body prevents the development of a scaly skin condition.

As a part of the diet, fats and oils from foods supply energy for body operation and bring with them the fat-soluble vitamins, nutrients that would be missing from the diet otherwise. The fatty foods also add variety to eating and may have a greater satiety value because they remain longer in the stomach than carbohydrate foods.

So, obviously, we ought not eliminate all fat from our diet. But we can pare it down, reducing calories—yet still getting enough for good health. To help implement this, some of the fat we ingest should be in the form of polyunsaturated fat.

In explanation, fat is said to be saturated if its molecules have all the hydrogen they can hold onto (saturated with hydrogen). But if the molecules can take on some hydrogen atoms, the fat is termed unsaturated; and if they can take on even more hydrogen atoms, the fat is called polyunsaturated, the prefix *poly,* of course, meaning "many." Most solid fat, such as animal fat, is saturated; but most oils, like vegetable oils, are polyunsaturated. (An oil is a fat that is liquid at room temperature.)

Polyunsaturated fat is emphasized in the diet for two reasons: it generally contains linoleic acid, a material which the body must have but cannot manufacture itself; and because it lowers cholesterol in the blood stream.

Cholesterol, a waxy alcohol found in animal fat, has been implicated as a factor in arteriosclerosis (hardening of the arteries). But despite this strongly suspected connection, some cholesterol is absolutely necessary to the body for proper functioning. For instance, cholesterol is turned into vitamin D by sunlight. Also, bile fluids formed by the liver to aid in digestion are derived from cholesterol. And about one-sixth of the brain is composed of cholesterol. In fact, cholesterol is so important that the body will manufacture it if intake is stopped.

However, you can cut down and still be safe.

Overabundance of fat in the diet, besides providing too much cholesterol and too many calories, can also cause diarrhea and a type of skin rash.

The Food and Nutrition Board does not specify a definite RDA for fat because of the great variation in consumption that is still harmonious with good health.

Good sources of polyunsaturated fat, the kind we seek, come from the vegetable kingdom: corn oil, peanut oil, and safflower oil. Some margarines are also good.

The diet plans in Chapters Fifteen and Sixteen are low in fat, so that the dieter may supplement his meals with fat-containing foods in accordance with the instructions given.

PROTEIN

Amino acids are simple chemical compounds made up of carbon, hydrogen, oxygen, and nitrogen; when they link together in the hundreds and even thousands, many times with sulfur and sometimes with other elements, amino acids form the giant molecules of *protein*, the third class of energy nutrient.

The large number of amino acids (over twenty) and the various sequences in which they can be joined to one another in a protein molecule make the number of different kinds of proteins almost infinite. Because of this great variety in type and construction, it's not surprising that proteins are the most versatile of all food molecules and are called upon to perform hundreds of tasks in the human body—besides supplying energy, a function they usually relinquish to carbohydrates and fats.

Some of the jobs proteins do: the protein hemoglobin carries oxygen via the blood stream to the cells; insulin, one of the smallest of proteins, regulates blood-sugar level; another protein, keratin, is the basic constituent of hair and nails; muscles also rely primarily on protein for their makeup.

Since protein is constantly lost and degraded in the human system, replenishment from dietary sources is always required. What happens if the body does not receive enough protein? Without this vital nutrient, the body quickly deteriorates, becoming emaciated and anemic as hemoglobin is not replaced. If calorie intake is also low, protein from the tissues is cannibalized for energy, contributing to further atrophy. And if the deficiency continues, the final result is death. In children, when they survive, diminished amounts of protein lead to stunted growth and damaged brains.

Lack of protein in the diet is the world's number-one nutritional problem and is felt especially hard in the poorer nations where protein-containing food, because of the cost, is unavailable to the general populace.

However, we in the United States are more fortunate—with our abundant wealth and resources. The RDA of 56 grams (gm) of protein per day for men and 46 gm for women is met by the average American's daily food consumption. (An RDA for protein is set because the body must have a minimal amount of nitrogen, which the protein contains, daily to offset wasting of the tissues. Of course the RDA represents more than the minimum requirement, having as it does a built-in cushion.)

Dieters, on the other hand, must watch their protein intake, and must be concerned with more than just the total amount of protein they consume each day. The source of protein is also important. Here's why:

Of the twenty-plus amino acids that make up the various proteins, eight are necessary for life. Actually, the body needs more than these eight; but if a high enough quantity of the eight essential amino acids is eaten, the body can then manufacture from them the others it requires. Tryptophan, our old friend the precursor of niacin, is one of the eight.

Now, any food source of protein which has these eight essential amino acids in the right amounts—enough so that they can be made into the others—is said to be *complete;* complete, that is, in the sense that it offers the eight amino acids from which all others necessary for body functioning can be synthesized.

These eight have to be present at one time for the manufacture of the others to be possible; but not all foods which contain protein are complete.

Therefore, dieters who limit their selection of food in some manner run the risk of not receiving the right amino acids in the proper amounts.

It follows, then, that any diet plan pursued should include at each meal foods that are complete in protein, such as meat, the richest source of protein, or provide foods that when eaten together supply all of the essential amino acids. (Plant proteins tend to be incomplete. So anyone on a vegetarian diet who does not use milk or eggs—which are complete—in his regimen should eat a wide variety of plant-derived foods at each meal.)

The diet plans in Chapters Fifteen and Sixteen take all of this into account. They provide at least 55 gm of protein daily; and that's 9 gm more than the RDA for women and only 1 gm short of the RDA for men, which can be made up by the supplemental eating, a part of the overall reducing plan to be explained in the pages ahead. Most of the protein in the meals of the diet plans comes from sources already complete in this nutrient—so there is no problem obtaining the eight essential amino acids at one sitting.

Problems with protein can arise, however, if too much of this nutrient is ingested into the system, as is possible with the use of supplements.

Any extra amount of protein consumed beyond normal needs will have its nitrogen stripped from it and will be stored on the body as fat—a process which is the opposite of what dieters are trying to accomplish. Also, the nitrogen from this surplus protein will be excreted in the urine by the kidneys; and nitrogen can irritate these organs, something that can be harmful to the very young, the old, and the infirm.

So stick with regular foods selected wisely—it's the best way to get your protein.

PART TWO

Energy and Overweight

13

ON BECOMING FAT:
A HERITAGE FROM
THE CENTURIES

AN ESSENTIAL

The diet of a reducing plan, of course, must do more than provide all the nutrients in the right amounts necessery for good health; it must also encompass some mechanism for weight loss through the manipulation of food.

What is the correct approach?

Though many have been advocated, there is only one way that really works, a procedure based on a scientific principle that's been established by rigorous experiment.

To understand what it is and to employ it properly in a diet, we must first discover why people become fat in the first place—the actual cause of obesity. So, who or what then are the real villains behind overweight? Is it calories? Is it fat people themselves? Are they simply gluttonous, or weak-willed overeaters? Or are they victims of malfunctioning glands? Or what?

In reality, it's not any of these.

Let's hunt down the true culprits responsible for obesity. We begin our search with the concept of energy and how it relates to the accumulation of fatty tissue on the human body. After this we look into the brain; and then we take a step into the past and another into the future.

THE BASICS

To explain best the connection between energy and overweight, we will make use of an analogy. The functioning of the human body has often been likened to the workings of an automobile, and since this analogy for our case is a good one, as we saw in Chapter Two, we'll use this perhaps overworked comparison one more time.

First, energy. For our purposes we can think of energy as the capacity to do work and induce motion, and as having the capability to generate light and/or heat. Energy is the prime mover of the universe. It makes everything go. Nuclear energy causes the sun to shine. Radiant energy from the sun warms the earth. Electrical energy runs our appliances. And energy, too, is no less the driving force behind automobiles and human beings.

The family car chugs from one place to another by exploiting the chemical energy stored in the gasoline it carries in the fuel tank. To utilize this potential energy, the gasoline is first brought from the tank—by the fuel pump—to the carburetor, where it is mixed with air. This air-gasoline mixture is then sprayed into the piston chambers, the cylinders, and is there ignited by a spark. The resulting quick combination of air molecules with gasoline molecules causes energy to be released in the form of heat, and this heated mixture, expanding rapidly, pushes against the pistons. In sequence, the pistons rotate the drive shaft, which, through a series of gears in the transmission and the rear end, is linked to the wheels. The wheels turn—and down the road the old clunker goes.

The human body also uses chemical energy to function.

But it relies on food in three forms—carbohydrates, fats, and proteins—instead of gasoline as its source of energy. Oxygen molecules extracted from air taken in by the lungs combine chemically with food molecules to release energy in the living cells of the body. These food molecules are "burned" to provide energy as surely as the molecules of gasoline in your car are burned—only in a much slower and more controlled manner than the explosive liberation of energy in the cylinders of an automobile engine. The energy derived from food doesn't turn wheels but is used to contract muscles, maintain the functioning of organs, and so forth.

Now then, just as we are able to measure volume in gallons,

distance in miles, and temperature in degrees, we can also measure amounts of energy—whether it is contained in gasoline or in food. Energy is measured in units called *calories*. A calorie is the quantity of energy required to raise the temperature of one kilogram of water (2.2 pounds) one degree centigrade. A pound of gasoline releases about 5000 calories when combined with air and ignited. In other words, if we burned a pound of gasoline under 5000 kilograms of water in ideal conditions, the temperature of the whole mass of water would rise one degree centigrade, a calorie for each kilogram of water. A pound of fat, on the other hand, produces 3500 calories when burned and would raise the temperature of the same mass of water only about three-fifths of a degree. And protein and carbohydrates yield per pound only about half as many calories as fat—when energy is released.

The amount of calories consumed by a car and the human body can vary.

For instance, the car uses energy at a certain rate when it is idling: the engine is turning, the battery is charging, and all the gauges are working, even though the car isn't going anyplace. But if we drive the car over to Grandma's house, it will burn more gas, and hence use up energy at a greater rate.

Similarly, our bodies consume energy when we are not in motion (lying in bed, say). The heart continues to pump blood, the glands secrete hormones, nerve impulses keep firing, and so forth. This low calorie expenditure corresponds to the idling of a car and has a name: *basal metabolic rate*. The basal metabolic rate of a woman who weighs 120 pounds is roughly 1340 calories per day. That is, if all she does the whole day is to rest in bed, she will still burn 1340 calories—her inner processes carrying on.

As driving the car to Grandma's house increases the amount of energy spent, so will exercise (movement) increase the rate at which the human body expends energy. If our 120-pound woman engages in average activity all that day, such as housekeeping, her energy expenditure will grow by about 660 calories, bringing her total daily energy output up to about 2000 calories.

Now with this knowledge of calories we can prod our automobile analogy just a little more and it will show us how and why fat tends to accumulate on the human body.

Suppose we drive the car to Grandma's house every day, and every day the car uses 12 gallons of gasoline. If we pump 12 gallons of gasoline into the tank at the gas station each day, we balance exactly the energy burned with the amount added to the tank, and all is fine—everything is the same as when we started for Grandma's. But if we add 13 gallons of gas to the tank each day and use only 12, then the tank will begin to fill up, adding weight, and our car will become heavier daily—by the weight of a gallon of gasoline. We're putting in too much energy for the amount of driving.

So with our 120-pound woman. If she expends 2000 calories a day but takes in 2350 food calories each day, she, too, will begin to gain weight—at the rate of a pound every ten days. Her system converts the excess energy (it matters not whether it came originally from protein, carbohydrates, or fat—see Chapter Fourteen) and stores it in the form of fat on her body, usually around the abdomen, buttocks, thigh area, though it may be deposited anywhere: face, neck, arms, chest, back, internal organs. It builds up.

What she is doing is eating too much.

The converse of our example is also true. If when driving the car we stop short of Grandma's house every day, the car will not burn all of the 12 gallons of gas it takes to get there; and if we continue to add 12 gallons of gas every day as before, the car will again gain weight—representing too little driving.

This is also valid for our 120-pound woman. If she cuts down her activities so that she expends only 1650 calories a day but perseveres in eating 2000 food calories daily, she will put on weight—at that rate of a pound every ten days. In effect, she is not exercising enough to compensate for the quantity of food she is ingesting.

Our analogy ends, and the conclusion we draw from it is that obesity comes from eating too much, exercising too little, or—I'm sure you'll find by playing with the gasoline and calorie figures on your own—a combination of both. This is not an earth-shaking revelation, but it's logical—and true.

Does this mean then that fat people *are* responsible for their state? Again, the answer is *no*. Man has an inherent mechanism that governs appetite in relation to activity, and as originally designed by nature it is very accurate in balancing the two; but in today's world, because of certain "villains," this mechanism is not operating efficiently.

THE APPESTAT

Near the center bottom portion of the brain, in the section called the hypothalamus, are two small areas known collectively as the *appestat*. (The term is derived from a combination of the word *appetite* and the Greek suffix *-stat*, which means "that which is regulated.") The appestat presides over our appetites much as a thermostat controls the temperature in our homes. The appestat shuts hunger on and off like the thermostat turns on and off the fire in a furnace.

Probably by sensing changes in blood chemistry, one of the tiny twin areas of the appestat tells us when we are hungry, and the other tells us when we've had enough to eat.

When our bodies require food for energy, the hunger portion sends to the conscious mind a message saying that we are hungry; at the same time it sends nerve impulses to the stomach, causing the stomach to contract rhythmically. These contractions give us a feeling of emptiness and make our stomachs growl. The result of all this is that we want to eat. Then, after we've consumed a certain amount of food, the other half of the appestat, the satiety portion, calls a halt to eating. The craving is ended, and we have a feeling of being full.

It is the appestat in the brain, and not the stomach, that controls hunger. Much of our knowledge of the appestat has come from scientific studies of animals—in particular, rats. Rats have appetite-regulating mechanisms similar to those found in humans, and experiments on them definitely show that it is the brain and nothing else that influences the feeling of hunger. For instance, when the hunger portion of a rat's appestat is surgically destroyed, the rat does not become hungry. It desires no food whatsoever, even though soon it is starving and would literally starve to death with food in reach if left unattended. Likewise, if the satiety portion of the rat's appestat is destroyed, the rat does not know when to stop eating and becomes hugely obese—to the point where it can hardly move.

We don't perform such experiments on humans, but on extremely rare occasions people have been known to suffer from lesions of the hypothalamus which damage the satiety portion of the appestat. These persons invariably become fat. As with the altered rats, they no longer know when to push themselves away from the table—they never have the sensation of being full. But these instances are quite infrequent, and though they confirm the role of the appestat in eating, they do not explain why the vast majority of overweight people, whose appestats are undamaged, are in that condition.

Part of the answer lies in the adjustment of the appestat itself. One of the functions of the appestat is to sense the rate at which the body expends energy, that is, how much we move, work, and exercise. But because the appestat evolved into existence back in primitive times, it is set to operate effectively at a much higher level of activity than is required by today's living, a level more appropriate to the hard life of the Stone Age, when long hours were spent just gathering food, finding shelter, and so forth. If we don't expend this amount of energy—and, of course, today most of us don't—the appestat in the brain doesn't function properly, and it consistently *overestimates* the quantity of food we should eat to balance our energy output. We ingest more food than we need before the hunger portion of the appestat shuts off our hunger pangs. Consequently, our waistlines expand.

This hypothesis has been confirmed with animal studies. Rats that are kept in cages too small for movement become fat when allowed to eat all they want. Other rats, permitted to exercise, eat only as much as they need to equalize their energy expenditures, even when unlimited amounts of food are made available to them.

So a mistuned appestat can take some of the credit for obesity in modern man.

But unlike the rat of the experiments, man is not confined to cages; he has every opportunity to exercise and reinstate the proper functioning of his appestat.

But we, the overweight, don't do it. We think about increasing our activity, but when we get right down to it, we put it off; we find we don't want to do any extra work—that we have an actual feeling of aversion for exercise. Why? If we were to exercise, not only would our appestats work better and limit our intake of food to what we need by controlling our hunger, but we would also improve our health and overall physical conditioning, and perhaps lead more productive lives.

It sounds so sensible and natural to exercise. What is it, then, that prevents us from extending our activity? Two things: progress, and an inheritance from our ancestors.

A BIRTHRIGHT TURNED SOUR

Today we live in an age of great technological advancement. We've built huge cities of steel and concrete. We've harnessed the awesome power of atomic energy. We've sent men to walk on the moon. And since the dawn of the Industrial Revolution, we've watched machines take over more and more of the work that man once had to do by the sweat of his brow. The machines perform our exercise for us. Where before we would have walked to our destinations, today we ride in automobiles; where before we would have washed clothes by hand, today we load them into automatic washers; where before we had to do accounting by paper and pencil, today computers do it. And that's not bad! The machines have freed us from drudgery, from the time when every act was an act for survival and nothing else. But what the machines have also done is upset our energy balance. We're still programmed for the Stone Age when we had to expend large amounts of energy. Today, however, because of the machines, we don't burn so many calories; yet our bodies still take the energy from the food we eat and convert it to fat—in preparation for long and heavy activity that never comes. The fat accumulates, and we become overweight.

But, after all, human beings are pretty sensitive instruments fashioned for survival; instead of an antipathy for extra work, why don't we have some natural yen that would make us want to exercise and burn those now-superfluous and harmful calories?

We don't have that inclination because Stone Age man has left his descendants a legacy, one previously of great worth, but which today, by reason of the machine, is no longer useful, in effect now actually working against us.

You see, although the cave man was equipped for heavy energy expenditure, he was also lazy. This is not as contradictory as it might at first seem, for laziness among nature's creatures has a certain amount of survival value.

Take the lion, for example. We've seen lions on television; we've watched them chase down game on the African plains, using a lot of energy to obtain their food; but we've also seen that for much of the time they simply laze in the shade, exerting themselves only when they have to. Laziness helps them survive. How?

Suppose there is a maverick in a pride of these animals, a lion who is frisky by nature, who after his kill spends his time roaming over the veldt in search of fun and frolic while his companions lie under a tree taking life easy. Our lion will use up more energy romping around than will his fellows as they rest. This extra energy must come from somewhere, and, of course, it has to come from food. Because of his internal disposition to friskiness, our maverick must make an additional kill every so often above that of the remainder of the pride in order to satisfy his increased energy demands. Repeatedly, our lion must test his muscles, reflexes, and stamina to bring down game one more time than his fellows. Since life is dangerous in the wild and food scarce, with his supplementary forays our lion's chances of surviving are less than those of his naturally lazy brethren, who pit their skills against nature only a minimum number of times. Probability tells us then that in the fierce competition for the scant resources of this planet it will be the frisky lion who will perish and the lazy ones who will survive to reproduce others in their mold. This is survival of the fittest— meaning those best equipped to succeed in a certain environment.

In this case, what is true of lions is also true of men. During the Stone Age life was difficult and hazardous, and the people most likely to survive were those who exerted themselves enough to remain afloat, but did no more than that. And it is precisely these Stone Agers, the ones geared for high energy output but with a sense of conservation, who endured—to pass their genetic patterns down to us.

In fact, man has changed little in genetic makeup since the Stone Age. Take a cave man, a Cro-Magnon, clean him up and shave him, dress him in a business suit, and we could not tell him from a modern man on the way to his office. Exterior appearance is virtually the same—and so are internal constitutions.

So, along with physical appearance, the appestat, and the ability to store energy in the form of fat on the body, which most animals have, our Stone Age progenitors have bequeathed us this other inborn characteristic—a tendency toward inactivity.

This tendency is readily apparent in our everyday lives. We stay in bed in the morning as long as possible. We drive to the store rather than walk, looking for the closest possible parking space to the entrance. At home and elsewhere we don't stand if we can sit;

and we don't sit if we can lie down. We buy periscopic gadgets that allow us to view the television screen without lifting our heads from the couch and other gizmos that let us change channels without ever having to get up. And what little work is left to us will soon be usurped by more and newer machines. Technology marches on.

But, in a sense, this wonderful technology that has emancipated us from manual labor has become a curse. It takes advantage of our built-in inclination to do as little as possible; when confronted with work, we listen to ancestral voices, and we surrender, letting the machines step in. But because we don't expend the energy, our appestats miscalculate, we overeat, and our waistlines suffer.

We're not to blame for being obese—we're merely the victims of heredity and progress, the "villains" mentioned at the beginning of this chapter.

And we can't let technology off the hook quite yet. One of the greatest technological developments in the history of mankind is represented by the abundance of food available in the Unted States. Modern tractors, reapers, combines, chemical fertilizers, and a thorough understanding of plant genetics have helped to make America the breadbasket of the world. We feed our own population and one-quarter of the rest of the earth's people besides. Our supermarkets are filled with food. It's omnipresent. Few of us today have ever had to go hungry for very long, unlike people in Stone Age times when food was to be had only at a premium—the price of gathering it, growing it, or running it down. When food was scarce, it was impossible to become fat. Today, calories almost swarm around us, and the temptation is to partake of them—to excess.

THE NEW LOOK

But not all of us are fat.

There seem to be plenty of lean people about who apparently get no more exercise than those of us who are overweight. Why is this so? How is it that they have escaped this pervasive problem of obesity? Scientists believe the answer is linked to the correct operation of the appestat.

But precisely why the thin person's appetite-regulating

mechanism might work better than the fat person's is not yet clear. It may be that by a quirk of nature the thin person's appestat functions adequately at a low level of activity. Or it may be that he is a secret energy user, expending calories in great numbers by constant nervous movement: playing with the change in his pocket, nodding his head to an unheard tune, tapping his feet, stretching, and making a hundred other incessant movements that require energy. At this higher level of activity his appestat is more likely to perform its job of tailoring appetite to energy expenditure.

Whatever the truth, the thin person represents the wave of the future. Because he is thin, he has few of the fat person's medical problems; he is healthier and will live longer; his kind will compete more successfully than the overweight in the battle of life as it now seems to be unfolding.

Survival of the fittest. Thin people will predominate in the centuries to come.

But you can compete with them today.

You can, that is, if you know which of the numerous methods of weight reduction advanced over the years are bogus and which are valid. That information is in Chapter Fourteen—along with more about calories. Do the calories provided by the energy nutrients have the same or differing fat-producing capabilities? We build on the knowledge acquired in this chapter.

14

ON BECOMING THIN:
MAGIC AND SCIENCE

ABRACADABRA

It's easy enough to *gain* weight. As we saw in the last chapter, all you have to do is give in to your natural desire and take in more calories than you burn; and since the human system absorbs nearly all digestible material and stores the energy from it in preparation for possible hard times to come, the fat will pile up.

But what about reducing?

Of course, the above procedure can be reversed.

You merely tilt your energy balance in the other direction and ingest fewer food calories than you burn; to make up the difference, your body will call upon the fatty tissue it stored for just this occasion, the fat will be oxidized for its energy, and you will begin to lose weight.

To start this process, the necessary caloric deficit can be induced in three ways: keeping activity the same, you can decrease the amount of food you eat—dieting; keeping the quantity of food you eat the same, you can increase your activity—more exercise; or you can combine both methods—dieting and getting more exercise simultaneously.

At first glance, none of these ways seems appealing. They go against our natural bent. Isn't there some easier route to losing weight we can follow, some magic that will melt away the pounds without the inconvenience of dieting or the agony of exercise? Certainly many such schemes have been ballyhooed over the years. Let's look at a few of them to see if they have any merit.

The ideal way to lose weight would be to swallow a pill that would remove the fat from the body chemically and dispose of it through normal elimination channels. Unfortunately, no such substance is known. Every now and then, though, a "drug" reputed to have this property is introduced to the public with great fanfare. Soon, however, it fades into oblivion and is remembered only by the federal government, which seeks out the makers because of claims that amount to false advertising. These materials can be classified with the tablets that turn water into gasoline, another fraud that occasionally peeks its head out from the land of legend and flim-flam.

Injections seem to have an even more powerful allure than pills. A current favorite is HCG, a hormone extracted from the urine of pregnant women. HCG injections are offered at many so-called "weight control clinics" run by medical doctors. A series of shots of this "fat mobilizer" may cost as much as $1000. Accompanying the HCG is a strict 500-calories-per-day diet. Of course, a plan like this would result in loss of three or four pounds a week in any case, even if the HCG had absolutely no effect. And its influence on obesity is questionable at best. A scientific study has shown that test subjects, when given injections of salt water, lose just as much weight on their restricted diets as when given shots of HCG. And salt water is much less expensive! Side effects of HCG have yet to be established.

Other drugs tried for weight reduction produce conditions more dangerous than the original one of obesity. Thyroid hormone falls into this category. In the past it was used in an attempt to raise the basal metabolic rates of some fat people in hopes that they would "burn up" more calories. But like most of the overweight, they already had thyroid glands that secreted a normal amount of hormone; and the extra-large quantity they had to take to increase their "idling speeds" upset their body chemistry, bringing on nervousness, excessive perspiration, insomnia, fatigue, fast pulse beat, and high blood pressure. Clearly, the medical risks were too great. And what weight the subjects did lose was immediately regained when administration of the drug was halted.

Another class of drugs that can be included in the dangerous group are the amphetamines. Popularly known as "diet pills" to the public, and as "speed" and "uppers" to the drug culture, these drugs were once widely employed to suppress appetite. But tolerance to them builds quickly, and the suppressing effect wears off in a week or two. Unless more and more are taken, appetite continues to return. But with such high dosage, amphetamines induce a dangerous, "hyped" mental state and often lead to strong psychological addiction. Like drugs of the heroin class, they are much abused. And as in the experiments with thyroid hormone, whatever weight is lost is gained back when usage is ended.

One type of drug which actually does cause weight loss, and which is relatively safe, is the diuretic. But there is a drawback: diuretics remove water from the body, not fat. And the weight loss in itself is only temporary, since sooner or later, to stay alive, you must drink back enough liquids to cover the deficit.

Some day science may produce a drug that will help in the fat-reduction process; but it is not yet here, and until the time comes when one is completely accepted by the scientific and medical communities as being safe, you're wise to stay away from any sort of wonder pill or injection.

Not all "miracles" that appear in the dieting world are dangerous, however; many are safe—they just don't work.

A few years ago an enzyme in grapefruit was hailed as performing the very desirable function of "burning up" any fattening foods you happened to eat and thus would subtract calories from your diet. All you had to do was eat lots of grapefruit after your meals, at which time the enzyme in the grapefruit would be released to go to work on the fat. Hence, the attractiveness of the eat-all-you-want grapefruit diet.

But the claim is fallacious. For one thing, there are no enzymes in grapefruit that will dispose of fat; for another, what enzymes do exist in the fruit work only in grapefruits and not in humans; lastly, grapefruit enzymes are digested in the human stomach with the rest of the fruit. People who stuffed themselves with food and then followed this act with massive amounts of grapefruit were chagrined to discover that they were gaining weight, and not losing it. Not surprising, since the enzyme is fictitious but the calories in grapefruit and the extra food are not.

Other methods touted for weight reduction bypass drugs, enzymes, and miracle potions altogether.

Two of these are the massage machine and the motorized exerciser. "Rub off your pounds" and "exercise your fat away" are the ideas.

In reality, however, the proposition runs more like this: the machine does the work, the salesman keeps your money, and you keep your fat—slightly jiggled. You can't break down fat by pounding it, squeezing it, shaking it, or riding it away on a motorized bike. To balance your food intake and to spark your appestat into regulating your appetite, you have to burn the calories yourself. We know that machines already impose far too much on our laziness. Why let one victimize you yet another time?

In a quite different approach, some of the many remedies offered for obesity direct themselves to the limiting of total calorie consumption. On the market are certain bulk materials that contain few calories. You're invited to eat of them when you're hungry—in place of regular food. You load your stomach with them, you assuage your hunger pangs, and that feeling of emptiness disappears. You haven't ingested any calories, therefore you don't put on weight. Or so the advertisements would have us believe. They sound plausible, but after close examination these pronouncements prove to be only specious in quality.

For it's your appestat in your brain, and not your stomach, that controls hunger. The feelings from the stomach are simply a product of the appestat's actions. You can fill yourself with cellulose gelatin, sawdust, or cement, but if you haven't also taken in many food calories, you appestat will sense this and continue to demand that you do. That feeling of hunger just won't cease. If bulk material could deceive the appestat, then our Stone Age ancestors, whenever they'd failed to find food, could have eaten leaves, bark, and grass to alleviate the sensation of hunger and could have gone on comfortably through life until they starved to death, all the while thinking they were full. With the result that we wouldn't be here today to worry about obesity—or anything. Scientific appraisal aside, common sense tells us this method is not practicable.

There is one way to gorge yourself on real food and still avoid assimilating many calories. Through surgery, you can have your small intestine short-circuited. In this operation, a section of the small intestine is removed; once this has been done, food passes through the digestive system before it has a chance to be properly absorbed. But again, your appestat knows when you are ingesting enough food calories to satisfy your body's needs. After this operation you are not getting the right amount of nutrients and energy, and no matter how much you eat, your appestat will send you a message of constant hunger, a miserable condition to endure. Also, this form of surgery has a high mortality rate; and when it is successful, it's usually irreversible. You might not like the final effect, but the change is permanent.

A CALORIE BY ANY OTHER NAME . . .

Sometimes in the search for solutions to the problem of obesity, reducing magic is sought in the manipulation of the three food types we consume for energy—carbohydrates, fat, and protein.

Two of the most popular diet plans rely on this approach. Dr. Irwin Stillman in *The Doctor's Quick Weight Loss Diet* advises us that if we eat all the high-protein foods we want and nothing else, we will lose weight. He bases his plan on a phenomenon that occurs in the body called *specific dynamic action*, or SDA for short.

SDA, a well-known effect, is the extra energy employed by the body to digest food—with the complex molecules of protein requiring a little more energy to be broken down than the simpler ones of fats and carbohydrates. In other words, digesting food takes energy, with protein costing more than fats or carbohydrates.

Now, according to Dr. Stillman's reasoning, if you eat exclusively high-protein foods, to pay for the higher SDA of their digestion, your body will have to appropriate energy for the process from its store of fat; consequently, body fat will be burned, and you will lose weight.

There are, however, several inherent defects in the total concept—if not in Dr. Stillman's logic. First, though it does exist, the SDA effect in reality is small, even for a diet of *pure* protein; and for the consumption of the ordinary high-protein foods that Dr. Stillman recommends, it is utterly negligible, because normal foods always contain a mixture of the food types. Meats, for instance, which have greater amounts of protein than other foods, also have significant quantities of fat, much of it visible to the naked eye, but about 10 percent spread indistinguishably throughout the meat and impossible to separate. Try as we might, then, we cannot segregate protein; and with the proportion of protein always reduced by the presence of the other food types, the SDA for it, small to begin with, becomes too microscopic to be important.

But the *coup de grace* to Dr. Stillman's diet, in which you eat all you desire of his high-protein foods, is the functioning of the appestat. The appestat senses energy requirements and adjusts the appetite to meet them. When energy expenditure is heightened, and it doesn't matter whether it comes from an increased waving of your arms or from the SDA effect, the appestat will expand the appetite to cover the energy loss. So even if the SDA effect were large, which it isn't, you would merely eat more food to balance it—and you would never lose weight.

The second of the popular diet plans that seeks diet magic in the manipulation of the three food types is the one presented in *Dr. Atkins' Diet Revolution*.

In his book Dr. Atkins explains that it is not the entirety of caloric intake that counts in weight control but rather the source of the calories, stating that calories from carbohydrates are more fattening than calories from protein or fat. What is more, he goes on, by depriving the human system of carbohydrate calories to burn for energy, the body must turn to the energy stored in its fatty tissue; thus, body fat will be "mobilized"—and the result for the dieter will be pounds lost. "All calories are not equal" is his premise—as it has been the premise of a long line of people promoting low-carbohydrate diets.

And the amazing part about it is that you actually do lose weight in dramatic fashion when you go on a low-carbohydrate regimen.

Then are Dr. Atkins and the others right about calories? Do they really count? Do they have different values? Can we eat all we wish of certain foods and still lose weight?

The debate over calories and carbohydrates has gone on for years. Several short-term scientific studies of dieting are often cited to support the claim that calories from carbohydrates are more fattening than calories from the other food types. In these studies, volunteers who were placed on low-carbohydrate diets did lose weight faster than others on high-carbohydrate diets of the same number of calories. From this, the experimenters directing the studies concluded that not all calories are equal. But they were misled—by time. The faster weight loss they observed is real enough, but their conclusion about how and why it happens is wrong.

A later study disclosed the truth. This definitive work on calories was done by Dr. Walter M. Bortz, Paula Howat, and Dr. William L. Holmes and was presented in the November 1968 issue of the *American Journal of Clinical Nutrition*. The study was conducted at the Metabolic Ward of the Lankenau Hospital in Philadelphia, lasted several months, and involved nine subjects: four women and five men, all but two of whom weighed over 300 pounds at the beginning of the experiment.

For alternating twenty-four-day periods each subject was fed exclusively one of two 800-calorie liquid diets daily. The diets were made up of carefully measured portions of carbohydrates, fat, and protein. But one diet contained zero carbohydrates while the other was high in carbohydrates. Protein content in both was the same. The study was tightly controlled, exercise in the ward regulated, and body weight recorded on charts to show weight loss versus time. At the end of each twenty-four-day period, the subjects were switched from one diet to the other and the experiment continued on the same controlled basis.

A second round similar to the first ensued—with sodium now added to both diets and the time periods lasting twenty-four and forty-eight days.

At the start of the project the researchers hypothesized that if calories were not equal in their fattening abilities, then the charts would show a different rate of weight loss for each of the two diets. But at the end of the first round of the experiment the rates were identical. Reduction was *not* any faster on the low-carbohydrate diet.

We can see this effect in Figure 1, the chart for one of the subjects. Except for small fluctuations in weight due to fluid loss and gain, the graph is a straight line with the same slope for both diets, indicating that the rates did not vary.

Marking this, the researchers concluded that it is the *total*

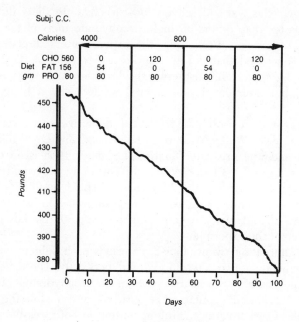

FIGURE 1*

*Used by permission of the American Journal of Clinical Nutrition

caloric differential that counts in weight reduction and not the composition of the diet. Carbohydrate, fat, and protein calories all have equal value.

But what about the earlier studies?

When the Philadelphia researchers resumed the experiment with sodium added to the diets in the form of table salt, they were able to duplicate the initial faster rate of weight loss with the low-carbohydrate diet that had showed up in the other studies. But because of the information obtained in the first round, they were able to demonstrate that the weight reduction came from the loss of water, not fat. Carbohydrates help retain sodium in the body, and when they are not present, such as in a low-carbohydrate diet, the sodium is excreted from the body in the water in which it is dissolved. Figure 2 illustrates this effect. This chart is of the same subject in Figure 1 after his diet was supplemented with sodium—to

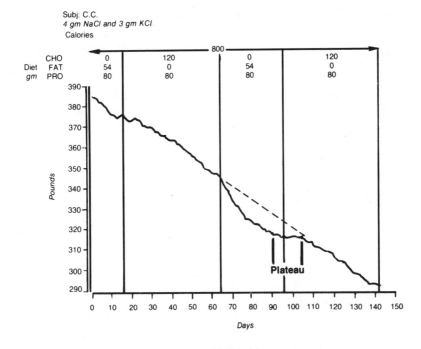

Subj: C.C.
4 gm NaCl and 3 gm KCl
Calories

			800		
CHO	0	120		0	120
Diet FAT	54	0		54	0
gm PRO	80	80		80	80

FIGURE 2*

*Used by permission of the American Journal of Clinical Nutrition

reproduce the more normal conditions of the previous experiments in reducing where salt was present in the diet.

Note in Figure 2 the initial rapid drop in weight after the subject switched from the high-carbohydrate diet to the zero-carbohydrate diet. Without the carbohydrates to retain sodium, his body at this juncture excreted the mineral in the water which contained it. This first drop, then, is largely water loss. Note now the leveling off in weight after the first drop. This is the diet "plateau" that is so discouraging to the people who try low-carbohydrate plans. Water loss has stopped, and weight reduction from this point on depends solely on the calorie differential between eating and energy expenditure.

For the subject after this passage of time, the net result of the zero-carbohydrate diet for weight reduction is the same as if he'd remained on the high-carbohydrate diet, where the rate of loss would have been slower but no plateau encountered, as indicated by the dotted line. The only difference during this period is the shifting of water weight, a diuretic effect, and of no real concern to the dieter.

If the studies carried out prior to the Philadelphia experiment had persisted beyond the water-excretion stage, they, too, would have demonstrated that in weight reduction it is the calories themselves that count and not their source.

There is no magic.

But there is science.

And science tells us that we can dispose of fat from our bodies simply by creating an energy imbalance: the number of calories we eat each day must be less than the number of calories we use up in daily living.

As we established at the beginning of the chapter, this situation can be achieved through dieting, increased activity, or a combination of the two.

Since exercise is anathema to most of us because of hereditary instincts we find difficult to deny, of the three methods *dieting* has the most appeal. We look at dieting in the next two chapters and put together all the knowledge we've gained into two diet plans.

Then in Chapter Seventeen we'll see whether or not exercise has any real value in weight reduction.

PART THREE

Reducing

15

HOW TO DIET: PLAN NUMBER ONE

OBSTACLES

What have we learned about dieting, nutrition, and energy?

In Chapter Two and the nutrient chapters we discovered that the body has an incontestable need for vitamins and minerals in the proper amounts—enough of these nutrients but not too much—and that getting them in just the right quantities when we diet can be tricky, with penalties to health and appearance if we make a mistake. And from the chapter on the energy nutrients we found out that dieting can be medically dangerous if the carbohydrate, fat, and protein content of the diet is knocked out of balance by emphasis on any one of them at the expense of those remaining. Chapters Thirteen and Fourteen demonstrated that unfortunately, despite our yearning for some magic which would dissolve away the pounds, calories do indeed count, a principle that cannot be ignored. Also, Chapter Fourteen showed us that we want to lose fat and not water. Yet, as we're confronted with all these difficulties, we still face the task of losing weight.

Can a diet plan be constructed and implemented that is safe and at the same time effective?

Yes—in fact, this book presents two of them, one carefully formulated by hand computation and described in this chapter, and the second devised with the aid of a modern digital computer and explained in Chapter Sixteen. Both diet plans incorporate all that nutritional science and medicine have learned about the problem of weight reduction. They use normal, everyday food that you purchase in the supermarket; and the menus evolved are constructed in accord with average American eating habits—with a little less emphasis on fatty foods and a greater reliance on green leafy vegetables of high nutritional and fiber content. Also, the diet plans embrace great variety and flexibility; you'll be able to enjoy your favorite foods, and your dieting will not become monotonous. Finally, the two diet plans in this book, founded on the concept of minimum calories, will give you all the vitamins, minerals, and other nutrients you need in RDA quantities or above. You won't be trading the problems of obesity for a profusion of other health hazards.

Let's take a look at the first plan.

HOW TO USE DIET PLAN NUMBER ONE

Because calories do count, the first step in utilizing Diet Plan Number One is to determine the total number of calories you burn each day. You do this quite easily by turning to pages 118–129 in this chapter. A glance at these tables shows us that daily caloric output depends on five different quantities: sex, age, height, weight, and amount of physical activity. Now, to ascertain your daily caloric expenditure, thumb through the tables until you locate the table and page that match your sex, age, and height. Then on that page run your finger down the left-hand column of figures under *Weight* until you find the weight, which is listed in pounds, that most nearly corresponds to your own. Now on that line move your finger across the page, stopping under the amount of daily physical activity that coincides with yours, which will be one of four classifications: *Light*, *Average*, *Moderately Heavy*, or *Heavy*. The number your finger is pointing to is your daily caloric expenditure, the figure for which we're searching.

You might have trouble deciding which of the four categories of physical activity applies to you. It depends on how you occupy your day. If most of your time is spent quietly sewing, or reading, or

watching television—in other words, moving around very little—
you would fall into the *Light* category.

But if your daily routine requires a little more effort, such as
working in an office, or driving a car, you come under the *Average*
activity column. Examples of people in this category are the average
housewife and homemaker, the average businessman, taxi drivers,
and most teachers and students.

However, if you're on the go most of the day, or if you participate in some form of recreation almost every night, then your activity is covered by the *Moderately Heavy* category. Door-to-door
salesmen, hospital nurses, housewives who keep large houses without the benefit of modern appliances, and those who play a few sets
of tennis every evening after work are in this classification.

People who engage in really exhausting physical labor are found
in the *Heavy* physical activity category. Examples include lumber-
jacks, coal miners, certain types of farmers, and athletes—such as
distance runners—who train long hours each day. But few persons
in this class have weight problems. The great amount of physical
exercise they perform allows the appestat, the appetite-control
mechanism in the brain, to function properly; and, of course, they
burn a considerable number of calories.

Now I would like to offer two cautions about determining your
calorie expenditure: First, the four categories of physical activity are
in no way related to the emotional or mental difficulty of your job;
they simply describe the amount of physical effort you expend during a day. For instance, the President of the United States, who has
one of the most demanding jobs in the world, would fall into the
Average or, at best, *Moderately Heavy* category. So choose accord-
ingly. The second caution is this: Don't exaggerate to yourself the
amount of physical work you perform during the day. For the diet
plan to operate successfully, you must select your correct daily
calorie expenditure number. So, if you really employ your hours
watching television, or sewing and reading, pick the *Light* category.
Or if most of your time is spent cleaning house, supervising the kids,
and going to market, choose the *Average* category. A point to remember: If you're contemplating a weight-reduction program,
chances are you fall into the *Light* or *Average* categories, in any
case.

Let's run through a quick example of how to use the calorie-expenditure tables. We'll suppose that you are a housewife, thirty-two years old, 5 feet 4 inches tall, with a weight of 137 pounds. We want to find your caloric output, so we flip through the tables until we come to page 119. This is the table for women between the ages of eighteen and thirty-six who are 5'2" to 5'5" tall. Now we look down the left-hand column, *Weight*, till we see the figure *135*, which is the number closest to your actual body weight. Next, since you're a housewife using modern appliances, we go across the page on that line to the *Average* category of physical activity. The figure in that column is 2127, your calorie-expenditure number. This means you burn approximately 2127 calories each day.

If you burn 2127 calories a day and eat 2127 calories of food during the same period, maintaining a steady fluid level, your body weight will remain the same. Eat more than 2127 calories and your weight goes up. Eat less, your weight goes down. A physical law, as we have seen in chapter Thirteen.

But how much less should you eat to lose weight safely? You could eat one calorie less each day and lose at the rate of one pound every ten years, which is obviously unsatisfactory because of the time element. Or you could fast, ingesting nothing, losing weight at the swiftest possible pace. But you would soon develop nutritional deficiencies and the associated diseases; and you would weaken yourself, thus becoming vulnerable to contagious disease and other medical liabilities we've discussed in previous chapters. So it's plain that fasting, too, is a poor method of dieting. The ideal calorie difference must lie somewhere between these two extremes.

What, then, is the optimum calorie differential?

To lose weight safely yet at a reasonable speed you should take in about 500 calories less each day than you burn. Why 500 calories particularly? An energy intake of about 500 calories less than you need daily will cause you to lose about a pound of fat a week. This might seem a slow pace compared to the claims of some of the diet plans foisted on the public; but it's a pound of fat you'll be discarding, not water; and over a year you'll shed 52 pounds—52 pounds that will stay off permanently. And you'll be comfortable. Yes, a greater calorie differential will cause you to lose weight faster; but studies have shown that you run the risk of ketosis, heart trouble, fatigue, and so forth, with a gap that's larger than 500 calories. A higher difference also means you'll develop a feeling of intense hunger. And hunger is a strong inducement to break a diet. So it's best to keep your intake about 500 calories below your daily expenditure. Go to a greater difference only with the consent of your doctor.

Now you have your calorie-expenditure number and you understand about the 500-calorie deficit for sensible weight reduction. The next step in Diet Plan Number One is to select your meals from the breakfast, lunch, and dinner menus that follow the calorie-expenditure tables in this chapter.

Looking through them, you can see that Diet Plan Number One is centered on a nucleus of thirty meals: ten breakfasts, ten lunches, and ten dinners, with the unique feature that any combination of any one breakfast, lunch, and dinner will give you at least the RDA for the essential nutrients. (Nutritional data for Diet Plan Number One are given on pages 150–153.) You'll never have to worry about them while dieting. They're built into the plan. You have only to concern yourself now with calories.

With that in mind, you choose as a single day's meals from the menus any one breakfast, any one lunch, and any one dinner—as long as the total number of calories in the three meals is 500 or more calories *less* than your calorie-expenditure number. And generally this gap will be greater than 500 calories. So you have a bonus—you can eat any foods you desire in addition to the meals chosen from the diet plan to bring the difference to about 500 calories, our safe limit. (The caloric value of over five hundred foods is listed in the Appendix for your convenience. Or you can use any of the calorie-counter books on the market.)

For clarity, let's return to the example of our housewife, whose calorie-expenditure number is 2127. She may choose for a day's meals any breakfast to go with any lunch to go with any dinner. Scanning the menus, she decides she will eat Breakfast No. 2 in the morning, Lunch No. 7 at noon, and Dinner No. 4 in the evening. The total number of calories for these three meals is 425 + 465 + 410 = 1300 calories. This is 827 calories short of her calorie-expenditure number of 2127 (2127 − 1300 = 827). Since she has to leave only about a 500-calorie gap, she has 327 calories to play with

(827 − 500 = 327); so she is free to eat 327 calories' worth of food beyond the three meals she has chosen from the diet plan. For instance, as an extra to her meals she might want to include three cups of black coffee, each with a teaspoon of sugar. Because coffee alone contains virtually no food energy, we do not have to worry about counting calories for it. The three teaspoons of sugar, however, contain a total of 40 calories (from the calorie listings in the Appendix) which we must tabulate. With her breakfast she might want to add two strips of bacon—90 calories. At dinner she might like a pat of butter on her baked potato—35 more calories for the butter. As a late-evening snack she may eat ten potato chips—115 calories. The total number of calories for this extra food is 40 + 90 + 35 + 115 = 280. This is within the 327-calorie limit with which she had to work. If she doesn't eat anything more that day, her net calorie deficit will be close to the 500-calorie difference between energy output and input for which we're shooting, calorie-expenditure number, of course, always being greater than calories consumed—by 500.

Note again that our housewife doesn't have to worry about the nutritional value of the extra food she eats beyond the three-meal core—just the number of calories. The RDA is always met by any combination of breakfast, lunch, and dinner she chooses. She will always get at least 55 gm of protein, 800 mg of calcium, 18 mg of iron, 4000 IU of vitamin A, 1.0 mg of thiamin, 1.5 mg of riboflavin, 13 mg of niacin, and 55 mg of vitamin C. These figures meet or exceed the 1974 Recommended Dietary Allowance for adult females. And her consumption of the additional foods will only increase them. She would be wise, of course, to avoid sugar altogether and limit foods high in saturated fats. Fat calories should provide no more than 30 percent of daily food energy intake.

The eating of favorite supplemental foods is not the only flexible aspect of the diet plan. You can have the meals in any order you like: lunch in the morning, a dinner at noon, a breakfast at night. Or you can interchange any foods among the three meals chosen. As long as you eat all of the food in a breakfast-lunch-dinner combination, your nutritional health is assured.

Many times you can fiddle with the meals themselves, as in the case of our housewife and Lunch No. 7—part of the meal calling for corned beef, lettuce, tomato, and a hamburger roll. She may eat each food separately, or she may make a sandwich of them, perhaps with a little mayonnaise. But she must remember to count the calories of any additions—one teaspoon of mayonnaise equals about 33 calories. This would bring her total calorie consumption for that day—including the calories in the sugar in the coffee, the bacon, the pat of butter, and the ten potato chips—to within 14 calories of our 500 calorie off-limits domain, which is all right.

Besides being flexible, Diet Plan Number One has great inherent variety. With ten breakfasts, ten lunches, and ten dinners there are $10 \times 10 \times 10$, or a thousand, different ways of arranging a day's meals. You could eat a new combination every day for the next two and a half years.

This variety and flexibility will help you to remain on your diet until you reach your weight-loss goal.

But you may want more discretion in the creation of individual meals themselves. If so, turn to Chapter Sixteen for a look at Diet Plan Number Two and how it simplifies this problem of foods, calories, and nutrition.

DAILY CALORIC EXPENDITURE — WOMEN

AGE: 18 TO 36   HEIGHT: 4´10´´ TO 5´ 1´´

PHYSICAL ACTIVITY

WEIGHT (LBS.)	LIGHT	AVERAGE	MODERATELY HEAVY	HEAVY
90	1415	1576	1732	1887
100	1509	1688	1861	2033
105	1555	1743	1924	2105
110	1600	1797	1987	2177
115	1645	1851	2049	2248
120	1689	1904	2111	2318
125	1733	1956	2172	2388
130	1776	2008	2233	2457
135	1818	2060	2293	2526
140	1861	2111	2353	2595
145	1903	2162	2412	2663
150	1944	2213	2472	2730
160	2026	2312	2589	2865
170	2107	2411	2704	2998
180	2186	2508	2819	3130
190	2264	2604	2932	3260
200	2341	2700	3045	3390
210	2418	2794	3156	3519
220	2493	2887	3267	3647
230	2568	2980	3377	3774
240	2642	3071	3486	3900
250	2715	3162	3594	4025
260	2787	3253	3702	4150

AGE: 37 TO 56   HEIGHT: 4´10´´ TO 5´ 1´´

PHYSICAL ACTIVITY

WEIGHT (LBS.)	LIGHT	AVERAGE	MODERATELY HEAVY	HEAVY
90	1334	1525	1690	1855
100	1422	1633	1816	2000
105	1464	1686	1879	2071
110	1506	1739	1941	2142
115	1548	1791	2002	2213
120	1589	1842	2063	2283
125	1629	1894	2123	2352
130	1669	1944	2183	2421
135	1709	1994	2242	2490
140	1748	2044	2301	2558
145	1787	2094	2360	2626
150	1826	2143	2418	2693
160	1902	2240	2533	2827
170	1976	2336	2648	2959
180	2050	2431	2761	3091
190	2123	2524	2873	3221
200	2194	2617	2984	3351
210	2265	2709	3094	3480
220	2335	2800	3204	3607
230	2405	2891	3313	3735
240	2473	2981	3421	3861
250	2541	3070	3528	3987
260	2608	3158	3635	4112

DAILY CALORIC EXPENDITURE — WOMEN

AGE: 57 TO 76   HEIGHT: 4´10´´ TO 5´ 1´´

PHYSICAL ACTIVITY

WEIGHT (LBS.)	LIGHT	AVERAGE	MODERATELY HEAVY	HEAVY
90	1249	1470	1646	1821
100	1330	1575	1770	1965
105	1369	1627	1831	2036
110	1407	1677	1892	2106
115	1446	1728	1952	2176
120	1483	1778	2012	2245
125	1521	1827	2071	2314
130	1557	1876	2130	2383
135	1594	1925	2188	2451
140	1630	1974	2246	2519
145	1666	2022	2304	2586
150	1701	2069	2361	2654
160	1771	2164	2475	2787
170	1839	2257	2588	2919
180	1907	2349	2700	3050
190	1974	2440	2810	3181
200	2040	2531	2920	3310
210	2105	2620	3029	3438
220	2169	2709	3138	3566
230	2233	2797	3245	3693
240	2296	2885	3352	3820
250	2358	2972	3459	3946
260	2420	3058	3565	4071

AGE: 18 TO 36   HEIGHT: 5´ 2´´ TO 5´ 5´´

PHYSICAL ACTIVITY

WEIGHT (LBS.)	LIGHT	AVERAGE	MODERATELY HEAVY	HEAVY
90	1472	1633	1788	1943
100	1568	1747	1920	2092
105	1615	1803	1984	2166
110	1662	1858	2048	2238
115	1707	1913	2112	2310
120	1753	1967	2175	2382
125	1797	2021	2237	2453
130	1842	2074	2299	2523
135	1885	2127	2360	2593
140	1929	2179	2421	2663
145	1972	2231	2481	2732
150	2014	2283	2541	2800
160	2098	2384	2660	2937
170	2180	2485	2778	3072
180	2261	2584	2894	3205
190	2341	2682	3010	3338
200	2420	2778	3124	3469
210	2498	2874	3237	3599
220	2575	2969	3349	3729
230	2651	3063	3460	3857
240	2727	3156	3571	3985
250	2801	3249	3680	4112
260	2875	3341	3790	4238

DAILY CALORIC EXPENDITURE — WOMEN

AGE: 37 TO 56   HEIGHT: 5' 2'' TO 5' 5''

PHYSICAL ACTIVITY

WEIGHT (LBS.)	LIGHT	AVERAGE	MODERATELY HEAVY	HEAVY
90	1391	1581	1746	1911
100	1481	1692	1875	2059
105	1524	1746	1939	2132
110	1568	1800	2002	2204
115	1610	1853	2064	2275
120	1652	1906	2126	2346
125	1694	1958	2188	2417
130	1735	2010	2248	2487
135	1776	2061	2309	2557
140	1816	2112	2369	2626
145	1856	2163	2429	2695
150	1896	2213	2488	2763
160	1973	2312	2605	2899
170	2050	2410	2721	3033
180	2126	2506	2836	3166
190	2200	2602	2950	3299
200	2273	2696	3063	3430
210	2346	2790	3175	3560
220	2417	2882	3286	3690
230	2488	2974	3396	3818
240	2558	3066	3506	3946
250	2628	3156	3615	4073
260	2696	3246	3723	4200

AGE: 57 TO 76   HEIGHT: 5' 2'' TO 5' 5''

PHYSICAL ACTIVITY

WEIGHT (LBS.)	LIGHT	AVERAGE	MODERATELY HEAVY	HEAVY
90	1306	1527	1702	1877
100	1389	1634	1829	2024
105	1429	1687	1891	2096
110	1469	1739	1953	2167
115	1508	1791	2015	2239
120	1547	1842	2075	2309
125	1585	1892	2136	2379
130	1623	1942	2196	2449
135	1661	1992	2255	2518
140	1698	2041	2314	2587
145	1734	2090	2373	2655
150	1771	2139	2431	2723
160	1843	2235	2547	2859
170	1913	2331	2662	2993
180	1983	2425	2775	3126
190	2051	2518	2888	3258
200	2119	2610	2999	3389
210	2185	2701	3110	3519
220	2251	2791	3220	3648
230	2316	2881	3329	3777
240	2381	2970	3438	3905
250	2445	3058	3545	4032
260	2508	3146	3653	4159

DAILY CALORIC EXPENDITURE — WOMEN

AGE: 18 TO 36   HEIGHT: 5˝ 6˝˝ TO 5˝ 9˝˝

PHYSICAL ACTIVITY

WEIGHT (LBS.)	LIGHT	AVERAGE	MODERATELY HEAVY	HEAVY
90	1528	1689	1845	2000
100	1627	1806	1979	2151
105	1675	1863	2045	2226
110	1723	1920	2110	2300
115	1770	1976	2174	2373
120	1816	2031	2238	2445
125	1862	2086	2302	2518
130	1907	2140	2365	2589
135	1952	2194	2427	2660
140	1997	2247	2489	2731
145	2040	2300	2550	2801
150	2084	2352	2611	2870
160	2170	2456	2732	3008
170	2254	2558	2852	3145
180	2337	2659	2970	3281
190	2419	2759	3087	3415
200	2499	2857	3202	3548
210	2579	2955	3317	3680
220	2657	3051	3431	3811
270	2735	3147	3544	3941
240	2812	3241	3656	4070
250	2888	3335	3767	4199
260	2963	3429	3877	4326

AGE: 37 TO 56   HEIGHT: 5˝ 6˝˝ TO 5˝ 9˝˝

PHYSICAL ACTIVITY

WEIGHT (LBS.)	LIGHT	AVERAGE	MODERATELY HEAVY	HEAVY
90	1447	1638	1803	1968
100	1540	1751	1934	2118
105	1585	1807	1999	2192
110	1629	1862	2063	2265
115	1673	1916	2127	2338
120	1716	1970	2190	2410
125	1759	2023	2252	2482
130	1801	2076	2314	2553
135	1843	2128	2376	2623
140	1884	2180	2437	2694
145	1925	2232	2497	2763
150	1965	2283	2558	2833
160	2045	2384	2677	2971
170	2124	2483	2795	3107
180	2201	2582	2912	3242
190	2277	2679	3027	3376
200	2352	2775	3142	3509
210	2426	2870	3255	3641
220	2499	2965	3368	3772
230	2572	3058	3480	3902
240	2643	3151	3591	4031
250	2714	3243	3701	4160
260	2784	3334	3811	4288

DAILY CALORIC EXPENDITURE — WOMEN

AGE: 57 TO 76   HEIGHT: 5´ 6´´ TO 5´ 9´´

PHYSICAL ACTIVITY

WEIGHT (LBS.)	LIGHT	AVERAGE	MODERATELY HEAVY	HEAVY
90	1362	1583	1759	1934
100	1448	1693	1888	2083
105	1489	1747	1952	2156
110	1530	1800	2015	2229
115	1571	1853	2077	2301
120	1611	1905	2139	2373
125	1650	1957	2200	2444
130	1689	2008	2261	2515
135	1728	2059	2322	2585
140	1766	2109	2382	2655
145	1803	2159	2442	2724
150	1841	2209	2501	2793
160	1914	2307	2619	2931
170	1987	2404	2735	3066
180	2058	2500	2851	3201
190	2128	2595	2965	3335
200	2197	2688	3078	3468
210	2266	2781	3190	3599
220	2333	2873	3302	3730
230	2400	2965	3413	3861
240	2466	3055	3523	3990
250	2531	3145	3632	4119
260	2596	3234	3741	4247

AGE: 18 TO 36   HEIGHT: 5´10´´ TO 6´ 1´´

PHYSICAL ACTIVITY

WEIGHT (LBS.)	LIGHT	AVERAGE	MODERATELY HEAVY	HEAVY
90	1585	1746	1901	2056
100	1686	1865	2038	2210
105	1736	1924	2105	2286
110	1784	1981	2171	2361
115	1833	2038	2237	2435
120	1880	2095	2302	2509
125	1927	2151	2367	2582
130	1973	2206	2430	2655
135	2019	2261	2494	2727
140	2065	2315	2557	2799
145	2109	2369	2619	2870
150	2154	2422	2681	2940
160	2241	2528	2804	3080
170	2328	2632	2925	3219
180	2412	2735	3045	3356
190	2496	2836	3164	3492
200	2578	2936	3281	3627
210	2659	3035	3398	3760
220	2739	3133	3513	3893
230	2819	3230	3627	4024
240	2897	3327	3741	4155
250	2974	3422	3854	4285
260	3051	3517	3965	4414

DAILY CALORIC EXPENDITURE — WOMEN

AGE: 37 TO 56   HEIGHT: 5'10'' TO 6' 1''

PHYSICAL ACTIVITY

WEIGHT (LBS.)	LIGHT	AVERAGE	MODERATELY HEAVY	HEAVY
90	1504	1694	1859	2024
100	1599	1810	1994	2177
105	1645	1867	2060	2252
110	1691	1923	2125	2327
115	1736	1979	2190	2401
120	1780	2034	2254	2474
125	1824	2088	2317	2546
130	1867	2142	2380	2619
135	1910	2195	2443	2690
140	1952	2248	2505	2762
145	1994	2300	2566	2832
150	2035	2353	2628	2903
160	2117	2455	2749	3042
170	2197	2557	2869	3180
180	2276	2657	2987	3317
190	2354	2756	3104	3453
200	2431	2854	3221	3588
210	2507	2951	3336	3721
220	2581	3047	3450	3854
230	2655	3142	3563	3985
240	2728	3236	3676	4116
250	2801	3329	3788	4246
260	2872	3422	3899	4376

AGE: 57 TO 76   HEIGHT: 5'10'' TO 6' 1''

PHYSICAL ACTIVITY

WEIGHT (LBS.)	LIGHT	AVERAGE	MODERATELY HEAVY	HEAVY
90	1419	1640	1815	1990
100	1507	1752	1947	2142
105	1550	1807	2012	2216
110	1592	1862	2076	2290
115	1633	1916	2140	2364
120	1674	1969	2203	2436
125	1715	2022	2265	2509
130	1755	2074	2327	2581
135	1795	2126	2389	2652
140	1834	2177	2450	2723
145	1872	2228	2511	2793
150	1911	2279	2571	2863
160	1986	2379	2691	3002
170	2060	2478	2809	3140
180	2134	2575	2926	3277
190	2205	2672	3042	3412
200	2276	2767	3157	3546
210	2346	2862	3271	3680
220	2415	2955	3384	3812
230	2483	3048	3496	3944
240	2551	3140	3608	4075
250	2618	3231	3718	4205
260	2684	3322	3829	4335

DAILY CALORIC EXPENDITURE — MEN

AGE: 18 TO 36   HEIGHT: 5′ 2′′ TO 5′ 5′′

PHYSICAL ACTIVITY,

WEIGHT (LBS.)	LIGHT	AVERAGE	MODERATELY HEAVY	HEAVY
130	1968	2425	2732	3040
140	2074	2566	2897	3227
145	2126	2636	2978	3321
150	2177	2705	3059	3414
155	2229	2774	3140	3506
160	2280	2842	3220	3598
165	2330	2910	3300	3690
170	2380	2978	3380	3782
175	2430	3046	3459	3873
180	2480	3113	3538	3964
185	2529	3180	3617	4054
190	2578	3247	3696	4145
200	2676	3379	3852	4324
210	2772	3511	4007	4503
220	2867	3641	4161	4681
230	2962	3771	4314	4857
240	3055	3899	4466	5033
250	3148	4027	4618	5209
260	3240	4154	4769	5383
270	3331	4281	4919	5557
280	3422	4407	5068	5730
290	3512	4532	5217	5902
300	3601	4656	5365	6074

AGE: 37 TO 56   HEIGHT: 5′ 2′′ TO 5′ 5′′

PHYSICAL ACTIVITY

WEIGHT (LBS.)	LIGHT	AVERAGE	MODERATELY HEAVY	HEAVY
130	1853	2343	2661	2980
140	1952	2480	2822	3165
145	2001	2548	2902	3257
150	2049	2615	2982	3349
155	2097	2682	3061	3441
160	2145	2748	3140	3532
165	2193	2815	3219	3623
170	2240	2881	3297	3713
175	2286	2947	3375	3803
180	2333	3012	3453	3893
185	2379	3077	3530	3983
190	2425	3142	3607	4072
200	2517	3271	3760	4250
210	2607	3399	3913	4427
220	2696	3526	4065	4603
230	2785	3652	4215	4778
240	2873	3778	4365	4953
250	2960	3903	4515	5127
260	3046	4027	4663	5300
270	3132	4150	4811	5472
280	3217	4273	4959	5644
290	3302	4395	5105	5815
300	3386	4517	5251	5986

DAILY CALORIC EXPENDITURE — MEN

AGE: 57 TO 76   HEIGHT: 5′ 2″ TO 5′ 5″

PHYSICAL ACTIVITY

WEIGHT (LBS.)	LIGHT	AVERAGE	MODERATELY HEAVY	HEAVY
130	1732	2257	2587	2916
140	1824	2389	2744	3100
145	1869	2455	2823	3191
150	1914	2520	2901	3281
155	1959	2585	2978	3372
160	2003	2650	3056	3462
165	2048	2714	3133	3551
170	2091	2778	3209	3641
175	2135	2842	3286	3730
180	2178	2905	3362	3819
185	2221	2969	3438	3907
190	2264	3032	3514	3996
200	2349	3157	3664	4172
210	2433	3282	3814	4347
220	2517	3405	3963	4522
230	2599	3528	4112	4695
240	2681	3650	4259	4868
250	2762	3772	4406	5040
260	2843	3893	4552	5212
270	2922	4013	4698	5383
280	3002	4133	4843	5553
290	3081	4252	4988	5723
300	3159	4371	5132	5893

AGE: 18 TO 36   HEIGHT: 5′ 6″ TO 5′ 9″

PHYSICAL ACTIVITY

WEIGHT (LBS.)	LIGHT	AVERAGE	MODERATELY HEAVY	HEAVY
130	2008	2465	2772	3079
140	2114	2607	2938	3268
145	2167	2677	3020	3362
150	2219	2747	3101	3456
155	2271	2816	3183	3549
160	2323	2885	3264	3642
165	2374	2954	3344	3734
170	2425	3023	3424	3826
175	2475	3091	3504	3918
180	2525	3158	3584	4009
185	2575	3226	3663	4100
190	2625	3293	3742	4191
200	2723	3426	3899	4372
210	2820	3559	4055	4551
220	2917	3690	4210	4730
230	3012	3821	4364	4908
240	3106	3950	4518	5085
250	3200	4079	4670	5261
260	3293	4207	4822	5436
270	3385	4335	4973	5611
280	3476	4461	5123	5784
290	3567	4587	5272	5958
300	3657	4713	5421	6130

DAILY CALORIC EXPENDITURE — MEN

AGE: 37 TO 56   HEIGHT: 5′ 6″ TO 5′ 9″

PHYSICAL ACTIVITY

WEIGHT (LBS.)	LIGHT	AVERAGE	MODERATELY HEAVY	HEAVY
130	1892	2383	2701	3019
140	1993	2521	2863	3206
145	2042	2589	2944	3299
150	2091	2657	3024	3391
155	2140	2724	3104	3483
160	2188	2792	3183	3575
165	2236	2859	3262	3666
170	2294	2925	3341	3757
175	2331	2991	3420	3848
180	2378	3057	3498	3938
185	2425	3123	3576	4029
190	2472	3188	3653	4118
200	2564	3318	3808	4297
210	2655	3447	3961	4475
220	2746	3575	4114	4652
230	2835	3703	4266	4829
240	2924	3829	4417	5004
250	3012	3955	4567	5179
260	3099	4080	4716	5353
270	3186	4204	4865	5526
280	3272	4328	5013	5698
290	3357	4451	5161	5870
300	3442	4573	5308	6042

AGE: 57 TO 76   HEIGHT: 5′ 6″ TO 5′ 9″

PHYSICAL ACTIVITY

WEIGHT (LBS.)	LIGHT	AVERAGE	MODERATELY HEAVY	HEAVY
130	1771	2296	2626	2956
140	1865	2430	2785	3140
145	1911	2496	2864	3232
150	1956	2562	2943	3323
155	2002	2628	3021	3414
160	2047	2693	3099	3505
165	2091	2758	3176	3595
170	2136	2822	3254	3685
175	2180	2887	3331	3775
180	2224	2951	3407	3864
185	2267	3015	3484	3953
190	2311	3078	3560	4042
200	2397	3204	3712	4219
210	2482	3330	3863	4395
220	2566	3455	4013	4571
230	2649	3578	4162	4745
240	2732	3701	4310	4919
250	2814	3824	4458	5092
260	2895	3946	4605	5265
270	2976	4067	4752	5437
280	3056	4187	4898	5608
290	3136	4307	5043	5779
300	3215	4427	5188	5949

DAILY CALORIC EXPENDITURE — MEN

AGE: 18 TO 36   HEIGHT: 5'10" TO 6' 1"

PHYSICAL ACTIVITY

WEIGHT (LBS.)	LIGHT	AVERAGE	MODERATELY HEAVY	HEAVY
130	2047	2504	2812	3119
140	2155	2648	2978	3309
145	2209	2718	3061	3404
150	2261	2789	3143	3498
155	2314	2859	3225	3591
160	2366	2929	3307	3685
165	2418	2998	3388	3778
170	2469	3067	3469	3870
175	2520	3136	3549	3963
180	2571	3204	3629	4054
185	2621	3272	3709	4146
190	2671	3339	3788	4237
200	2770	3474	3946	4419
210	2869	3607	4103	4600
220	2966	3740	4259	4779
230	3062	3871	4414	4958
240	3157	4002	4569	5136
250	3252	4131	4722	5313
260	3346	4260	4874	5489
270	3439	4388	5026	5664
280	3531	4516	5177	5839
290	3623	4643	5328	6013
300	3714	4769	5477	6186

AGE: 37 TO 56   HEIGHT: 5'10" TO 6' 1"

PHYSICAL ACTIVITY

WEIGHT (LBS.)	LIGHT	AVERAGE	MODERATELY HEAVY	HEAVY
130	1932	2422	2741	3059
140	2033	2562	2904	3247
145	2084	2630	2985	3340
150	2133	2699	3066	3433
155	2182	2767	3146	3526
160	2231	2835	3226	3618
165	2280	2902	3306	3710
170	2328	2969	3385	3802
175	2376	3036	3464	3893
180	2424	3103	3543	3984
185	2471	3169	3622	4074
190	2518	3235	3700	4165
200	2611	3366	3855	4345
210	2704	3496	4010	4524
220	2795	3625	4163	4702
230	2885	3753	4316	4879
240	2975	3880	4468	5055
250	3064	4007	4619	5231
260	3152	4133	4769	5405
270	3240	4258	4919	5580
280	3326	4382	5068	5753
290	3412	4506	5216	5926
300	3498	4629	5364	6098

DAILY CALORIC EXPENDITURE — MEN

AGE: 57 TO 76   HEIGHT: 5'10'' TO 6' 1''

PHYSICAL ACTIVITY

WEIGHT (LBS.)	LIGHT	AVERAGE	MODERATELY HEAVY	HEAVY
130	1811	2336	2666	2996
140	1905	2471	2826	3181
145	1952	2538	2906	3273
150	1998	2604	2985	3365
155	2044	2670	3064	3457
160	2090	2736	3142	3548
165	2135	2802	3220	3639
170	2180	2867	3298	3729
175	2225	2932	3376	3820
180	2269	2996	3453	3909
185	2313	3060	3530	3999
190	2357	3125	3607	4089
200	2444	3252	3759	4267
210	2530	3378	3911	4444
220	2615	3504	4062	4620
230	2700	3629	4212	4796
240	2783	3753	4361	4970
250	2866	3876	4510	5144
260	2948	3999	4658	5318
270	3030	4120	4805	5490
280	3111	4242	4952	5663
290	3191	4363	5098	5834
300	3271	4483	5244	6005

AGE: 18 TO 36   HEIGHT: 6' 2'' TO 6' 5''

PHYSICAL ACTIVITY

WEIGHT (LBS.)	LIGHT	AVERAGE	MODERATELY HEAVY	HEAVY
130	2087	2544	2851	3158
140	2196	2688	3019	3350
145	2250	2760	3103	3445
150	2303	2831	3185	3540
155	2356	2902	3268	3634
160	2409	2972	3350	3728
165	2461	3042	3432	3821
170	2513	3111	3513	3915
175	2565	3180	3594	4007
180	2616	3249	3674	4100
185	2667	3318	3755	4192
190	2718	3386	3835	4284
200	2818	3521	3994	4466
210	2917	3656	4152	4648
220	3015	3789	4309	4829
230	3112	3921	4465	5008
240	3209	4053	4620	5187
250	3304	4183	4774	5365
260	3399	4313	4927	5542
270	3492	4442	5080	5718
280	3586	4570	5232	5893
290	3678	4698	5383	6068
300	3770	4825	5534	6242

DAILY CALORIC EXPENDITURE — MEN

AGE: 37 TO 56   HEIGHT: 6´ 2´´ TO 6´ 5´´

PHYSICAL ACTIVITY

WEIGHT (LBS.)	LIGHT	AVERAGE	MODERATELY HEAVY	HEAVY
130	1972	2462	2780	3098
140	2074	2602	2945	3288
145	2125	2672	3027	3382
150	2175	2741	3108	3475
155	2225	2810	3189	3568
160	2275	2878	3270	3661
165	2324	2946	3350	3754
170	2373	3014	3430	3846
175	2421	3081	3509	3938
180	2469	3148	3589	4029
185	2517	3215	3668	4120
190	2565	3281	3746	4211
200	2659	3413	3903	4392
210	2752	3544	4058	4572
220	2844	3674	4213	4751
230	2936	3803	4366	4929
240	3026	3931	4519	5106
250	3116	4059	4671	5283
260	3205	4186	4822	5458
270	3293	4312	4972	5633
280	3381	4437	5122	5808
290	3468	4561	5271	5981
300	3554	4686	5420	6154

AGE: 57 TO 76   HEIGHT: 6´ 2´´ TO 6´ 5´´

PHYSICAL ACTIVITY

WEIGHT (LBS.)	LIGHT	AVERAGE	MODERATELY HEAVY	HEAVY
130	1851	2376	2705	3035
140	1946	2512	2867	3222
145	1993	2579	2947	3315
150	2040	2646	3027	3407
155	2087	2713	3106	3499
160	2133	2779	3185	3591
165	2179	2845	3264	3682
170	2224	2911	3342	3774
175	2270	2976	3420	3864
180	2314	3042	3498	3955
185	2359	3106	3576	4045
190	2403	3171	3653	4135
200	2491	3299	3807	4314
210	2578	3427	3959	4492
220	2665	3553	4111	4669
230	2750	3679	4262	4846
240	2834	3804	4413	5021
250	2918	3928	4562	5196
260	3001	4051	4711	5371
270	3084	4174	4859	5544
280	3165	4296	5007	5717
290	3247	4418	5154	5889
300	3327	4539	5300	6061

DIET PLAN NUMBER ONE

BREAKFAST # 1

Bacon	2 slices
Egg, cooked	1 egg
Milk, skim	1 cup
Peaches, cooked, unsweetened, and juice	$\frac{1}{2}$ cup
Orange juice	$\frac{1}{2}$ cup

430 calories

BREAKFAST #2

Egg, scrambled, milk added	1 egg
Special K cereal	1 oz.
Milk, whole	1 cup
Grapefruit	$\frac{1}{2}$ grapefruit

425 calories

BREAKFAST #3

Corned beef hash	3 oz.
Toast, white bread	1 slice
Yogurt made from skim milk, commercial, plain	1 cup
Tomato juice	1 cup

400 calories

BREAKFAST #4

Bacon	2 slices
Muffin, 3 in. diameter	1 muffin
Jelly	1 tbsp.
Wheaties cereal	1 oz.
Milk, skim	1 cup
Orange juice	$\frac{1}{2}$ cup

520 calories

BREAKFAST #5

Chipped beef	2 oz.
Egg, cooked	1 egg
Milk, skim	1 cup
Cantaloupe	melon

345 calories

BREAKFAST #6

Bacon	2 slices
Toast, white bread	1 slice
Margarine	1 pat
Cheerios cereal	1 oz.
Milk, whole	1 cup
Orange juice	1 cup

590 calories

BREAKFAST #7

Pork links	2 links
Toast, whole wheat	1 slice
Apricots, cooked	$\frac{1}{2}$ cup
Milk, skim	1 cup
Tangerine	1 tangerine

---

440 calories

BREAKFAST #8

Pork links	2 links
Yogurt made from skim milk, commercial, plain	1 cup
Maypo 30-Second Oatmeal	1 oz.
Apple	1 apple

---

430 calories

BREAKFAST #9

Chipped beef	2 oz.
Toast, whole wheat	1 slice
Yogurt made from skim milk, commercial, plain	1 cup
Orange juice	$\frac{1}{2}$ cup

---

365 calories

BREAKFAST # 10

Pancake, 4 in. diameter	1 cake
Syrup	1 tbsp.
Post Raisin Bran cereal	1 oz.
Milk, whole	1 cup
Grapefruit	$\frac{1}{2}$ grapefruit

425 calories

LUNCH # 1

Chicken, canned	3 oz.
Asparagus, canned	1 cup
Cheese, Swiss	1 oz.
Orange	1 orange

380 calories

LUNCH # 2

Tuna	3 oz.
Cheese, American	1 oz.
Bread, white	1 slice
Lettuce	4 leaves
Tomato juice	1 cup

415 calories

LUNCH # 3

Hamburger, lean	3 oz.
Hamburger roll	1 roll
Cheese, American	1 oz.
Lettuce	2 leaves
Tomato	$\frac{1}{4}$ tomato
Pickle, dill	1 pickle
Orange	1 orange

505 calories

LUNCH # 4

Stew, beef and vegetable	2 cups
Milk, skim	1 cup
Grapefruit	$\frac{1}{2}$ grapefruit

555 calories

LUNCH # 5

Hamburger, lean	3 oz.
Pickle, dill	1 pickle
Milk, skim	1 cup
Watermelon	1 wedge
Carrot	$\frac{1}{2}$ carrot

410 calories

LUNCH # 6

Salami	1 oz.
Bread, white	2 slices
Cheese, American	1 oz.
Lettuce	2 leaves
Pickle, dill	1 pickle
Tomato juice	1 cup

450 calories

LUNCH # 7

Corned beef	3 oz.
Hamburger roll	1 roll
Lettuce	2 leaves
Tomato	$\frac{1}{4}$ tomato
Milk, skim	1 cup
Plum	2 plums

465 calories

LUNCH # 8

Shrimp, canned	3 oz.
Bread, white	2 slices
Yogurt made from skim milk, commercial, plain	1 cup
Tomato juice	1 cup

420 calories

LUNCH # 9

Chipped beef	3 oz.
Bread, whole wheat	1 slice
Lettuce	2 leaves
Milk, skim	1 cup
Strawberries	1 cup

393 calories

LUNCH # 10

Clams, canned	3 oz.
French fries	10 pieces
Bread, whole wheat	1 slice
Milk, skim	1 cup
Strawberries	1 cup
Carrot	$\frac{1}{2}$ carrot

390 calories

DINNER # 1

Chicken, flesh, light meat	3 oz.
Potato, mashed, milk added	1 cup
Spinach, cooked	$\frac{1}{2}$ cup
Sauerkraut, canned	1 cup
Lettuce	2 leaves
Tomato juice	1 cup

360 calories

DINNER #2

Pork chop, lean meat only	1.7 oz.
Yellow beans, canned	1 cup
Cheese, Swiss	$\frac{1}{2}$ oz.
Bread, whole wheat	2 slices
Strawberries	1 cup
Carrot	1 carrot

430 calories

DINNER #3

Veal cutlet	3 oz.
Potato, boiled	2 potatoes
Dandelion greens	1 cup
Peach	1 peach

490 calories

DINNER #4

Steak, lean, broiled	2.4 oz.
Potato, baked	1 potato
Spinach, cooked	1 cup
Milk, skim	1 cup
Cantaloupe	$\frac{1}{2}$ melon

410 calories

DINNER #5

Chipped beef	3 oz.
Peas, cooked	$\frac{1}{2}$ cup
Lettuce	2 leaves
Carrot	$\frac{1}{2}$ carrot
Milk, skim	1 cup
Strawberries	1 cup

396 calories

DINNER #6

Ham, cured, roasted	3 oz.
Asparagus, canned	1 cup
Cheese, Cheddar	1 oz.
Peaches, cooked	$\frac{1}{2}$ cup

515 calories

DINNER #7

Hamburger, lean	3 oz.
Potato, mashed, milk added	1 cup
Spinach, cooked	1 cup
Orange	1 orange

415 calories

DINNER # 8

Shrimp, canned	3 oz.
Squash, summer	$\frac{3}{4}$ cup
Asparagus, canned	$\frac{3}{4}$ cup
Bread, whole wheat	2 slices
Lettuce	3 leaves
Peaches, sliced	1 cup

367 calories

DINNER # 9

Liver, beef, fried	2 oz.
Potato, baked	1 potato
Brussels Sprouts	1 cup
Cheese, Swiss	1 oz.
Orange	1 orange

445 calories

DINNER # 10

Oysters, raw	1 cup
Broccoli	1 cup
Bread, white	1 slice

270 calories

16

HOW TO DIET:
PLAN NUMBER TWO

THE MINIMUM-CALORIE DILEMMA

What is the very fastest way to lose weight?

This is a question often on the lips of potential dieters. In a sense it's a valid question and one that should be answered. We've talked about it before. To lose weight at a maximum rate, you must fast—that is, eat nothing, cutting calories to zero. Of course, fasting has drawbacks. You'll run into a host of problems, not the least of which are hunger and the diminishing supply of nutrients needed to keep the body healthy.

For the moment let's ignore the hunger and the medical troubles that occur with fasting and concentrate on the nutrition-versus-calories puzzle.

To lose weight quickly we want minimum calories, zero if possible; yet at the same time we must maintain an adequate supply of nutrients. For instance, we require about 55 gms of protein (RDA) every day for its invaluable nitrogen and tissue-building properties. But one gram of protein contains 4 calories; and an intake of 55 gms of pure protein each day—which we must have to thrive—means we automatically consume 220 calories daily, far above the zero we would like. And we still need other nutrients. But what if we were to choose the right food? Might we not get some of the other nutrients our bodies demand with our protein? And still keep calories to a minimum?

We'll start with calcium and milk. We know that milk is high in both protein and calcium. Drinking three large glasses of skim milk each day will give us 54 gms of protein, very near the RDA. Three glasses of skim milk also yield 1776 mg of calcium, over double the RDA for that mineral, so we're more than safe. But three glasses of skim milk contain 540 calories, quite a jump over our former minimum of 220 calories. And though milk is a good food, it contains very little iron, another necessary mineral. If we were to rely on skim milk to give us the RDA of 18 mg of iron, we'd have to drink 90 glasses of it a day, for a grand total of 16,200 calories! This, of course, is unthinkable. So we keep our skim milk at three glasses and add some oysters to our diet—oysters have lots of iron. But since oysters also possess some protein and calcium, we must decrease the amount of skim milk—to reduce total calories. So we subtract milk, calcium, and calories, and add protein and iron. But milk and oysters don't carry much in the way of vitamin C. Lima beans, however, do. But lima beans also contain some iron, calcium, protein— and calories. Because we don't want to increase the number of calories any more than we have to, we try juggling the three foods, their energy units, and their nutrients.

It's beginning to get complex. And we still have many nutrients to go. There are thousands of foods from which to choose, and we certainly don't want to eat oysters every day.

But we still want minimum calories, with all the nutrients, in reasonable amounts of the foods we enjoy. Whew!

The problem is so complicated that there might seem at first to be no solution at all. Fortunately, this is not the case. A way of solving problems like this was discovered by mathematicians in 1947. In fact, a whole field of mathematics has since grown up around the solution to such problems. This field is called *linear programming*, the word *linear* coming from the nature of the mathematics involved (having to do with straight lines, as in the graphing of linear equations), and *programming*, meaning the employment of a step-by-step method for solving the problem. A *program* is a particular procedure that is carried out to obtain the solution. This step-by-step method is easily implemented with an electronic computer, using a *computer program,* which is nothing more than a set of instructions telling the computer how to do the problem.

In actuality, we don't need the computer; the linear programming can be done by hand. But the computer is so much faster. To work out a group of foods which we like that contains minimum calories with the RDA for all nutrients would take hours and hours by hand. But the computer can do it in just 8.5 seconds! You can see the advantage, although using the computer does have some pitfalls. When I was first wrestling with the program that solves the minimum-calorie problem, I believed the computer would always come up with a reasonable number of servings of each food. I was wrong. When prompted to answer the calorie-nutrient question, the computer responded by saying that getting the RDA of essential vitamins and minerals with minimum calories was really quite simple: All you had to do every day was to eat—among a few other odd things—seventy-six stalks of celery! I made adjustments to the program.

But linear programming does give us exactly what we're looking for: maximum nutrition with minimum calories. Using the computer, we simply apply linear programming techniques to various combinations of foods.

And the sets of food assembled by the computer, which we'll call "food baskets," form the core of Diet Plan Number Two. Each of the ten food baskets, listed on pages 145–149, is the heart of a single day's eating and provides the RDA or better for the requisite nutrients—but always with minimum calories.

Diet Plan Number Two works in much the same way as Diet Plan Number One. First, you find your daily calorie expenditure number from the tables in the previous chapter; then, instead of choosing a breakfast, lunch, and dinner from Diet Plan Number One, you pick one of the ten food baskets of Diet Plan Number Two as your day's basic allotment of food. The idea again is to supplement the food basket, which will always furnish the RDA of the essential nutrients, with other foods you want—to bring the number of calories you consume to about 500 calories *below* your daily calorie-expenditure number. As in Diet Plan Number One, you'll lose about a pound of fat a week. True, if you eat only the food in the food basket, you'll lose weight at the maximum possible rate while still maintaining adequate levels of nutrition. But, as we have seen, this is not a wise choice, and you're urged to do this only under the supervision of your doctor. The real purpose of minimizing the number of calories in Diet Plan Number Two is to give you the widest possible latitude in selecting the supplemental foods you wish to eat. This leeway averts the rigors and monotony associated with other diet plans.

The housewife of our example appreciates this. With her calorie-expenditure number of 2127, she's shooting for a daily consumption of 1627 calories, 500 below the 2127. By selecting Food Basket No. 2 of 820 calories, she has 807 calories (1627 − 820 = 807) to make up by eating some of her favorite foods. So that day, besides the food in the food basket, she might eat a plate of spaghetti with meatballs and tomato sauce (two and one-third cups equal 770 calories) and six olives (about 30 calories) for a total of 800 more calories, very near the deficit of 807 calories it takes to raise her daily consumption to 1627 calories. On other days with the same food basket she may choose new foods to make up the difference. And there are nine more food baskets she might start with. You can see the scope this gives her—and you.

By the way, Diet Plans Number One and Two do not have to be followed separately. You can alternate them each day, or each week, etc., as long as you maintain that basic 500-calorie difference between intake and expenditure.

But whatever way you use the two diet plans, you'll have great variety, and you'll never have to worry about your nutritional health. That's locked into both plans.

LOOKING AHEAD

As you continue dieting, weigh yourself once every five days on the bathroom scale; and from your new, lower body weight you should locate your new calorie-expenditure number from the tables and re-figure your calorie intake, so that your intake remains 500 calories below the amount you burn each day.

Once you've reached your goal, you'll still have to tally

calories—to make sure you ingest only as many calories as you expend. But by now you are calorie-conscious, and you won't have any trouble with this. Keeping track of vitamins and minerals, however, without a computer or a pocket calculator is another story. What should you do about them? The best way to insure that you are getting enough of the essential nutrients is to prepare your meals from a wide selection of food. With every meal—or at least during the period of one day—try to include some foods from each of the different food groups: eggs and dairy products, meat and fish, vegetables, cereal, fruit. Variety is one of the keys to nutritional well-being.

This ends our discussion of dieting in relation to weight reduction. But there is another important factor that influences weight control—and you should have an understanding of it. We talk about exercise in Chapter Seventeen.

DIET PLAN NUMBER TWO

FOOD BASKET #1

Luncheon meat, ham	3 oz.
Bread, whole wheat	4 slices
Liver, beef	3 oz.
Spinach, cooked	$\frac{3}{4}$ cup
Milk, skim	2 cups
Cantaloupe	$\frac{1}{2}$ melon
Apple	1 apple

1002 calories

FOOD BASKET #2

Buc Wheats cereal	$1\frac{1}{2}$ oz.
Milk, skim	3 cups
Pork chop	1 chop
Peas, cooked	1 cup
Lettuce	2 leaves

----

820 calories

FOOD BASKET #3

Oysters raw, meat only	1 cup
Peas, cooked	1 cup
Cheese, Swiss	2 oz.
Lettuce	4 leaves
Bread, white	3 slices
Banana	1 banana
Ice cream, regular	1 cup
Carrot	$\frac{1}{2}$ carrot

1070 calories

FOOD BASKET #4

Bacon	2 slices
Total cereal	1 oz.
Milk, whole	3 cups
Tuna	3 oz.
Kale	$\frac{1}{2}$ cup

865 calories

FOOD BASKET #5

Chipped beef	3 oz.
Egg, cooked	1 egg
Peaches, cooked, unsweetened, and juice	$\frac{1}{2}$ cup
Heart, beef, braised	3 oz.
Collards	$\frac{1}{2}$ cup
Milk, skim	$1\frac{3}{4}$ cups
Toast, white bread	2 slices
Tomato juice	$1\frac{1}{2}$ cups

915 calories

FOOD BASKET #6

Bacon	4 slices
Product 19 cereal	1 oz.
Milk, skim	3 cups
Hot dog	1 dog
Pizza, $\frac{1}{8}$ of 14-in. pie	1 slice
Pear	1 pear

1015 calories

FOOD BASKET #7

Chipped beef	3 oz.
Cantaloupe	$\frac{1}{2}$ melon
Tomato juice	1 cup
Carrot	$\frac{1}{2}$ carrot
Bread, white	2 slices
Spaghetti, canned, tomato sauce and cheese	$\frac{2}{3}$ cup
Spinach, cooked	$\frac{3}{4}$ cup
Mushrooms, canned	$\frac{1}{2}$ cup
Lettuce	2 leaves
Pickle, dill	1 pickle
Milk, skim	$1\frac{1}{2}$ cups
Orange	1 orange

852 calories

FOOD BASKET #8

Corn muffin	1 muffin
King Vitaman cereal	1 oz.
Banana	1 banana
Chicken	$\frac{1}{2}$ breast
Rice, white, instant	$\frac{2}{3}$ cup
Broccoli	$\frac{3}{4}$ cup
Bread, white	2 slices
Carrot	1 carrot
Lettuce	2 leaves
Milk, skim	2 cups

990 calories

FOOD BASKET # 9

Egg, scrambled, milk added	2 eggs
Bread, whole wheat	4 slices
Peaches, cooked, unsweetened, and juice	$\frac{1}{2}$ cup
Bean with pork soup	2 cups
Steak, round, lean only	2.4 oz.
Asparagus, canned solids and liquids	$\frac{1}{2}$ cup
Sauerkraut, canned	$\frac{2}{3}$ cup
Lettuce	2 leaves
Milk, skim	$1\frac{1}{4}$ cup

1240 calories

FOOD BASKET # 10

Peanut butter	1 tbsp.
Bread, white	2 slices
Total cereal	1 oz.
Milk, skim	$2\frac{1}{2}$ cups
Lamb chop, broiled	1 chop

---

980 calories

NUTRITIONAL DATA
FOR DIET PLANS
ONE AND TWO

The following abbreviations are used:
cal: calories
mg: milligrams
IU: International Units

Diet Plan Number One
Nutritional Data

		ENERGY (cal)	PRO-TEIN (grams)	CAL-CIUM (mg)	IRON (mg)	VITAMIN A (IU)	THIAMIN (mg)	RIBO-FLAVIN (mg)	NIACIN (mg)	VITAMIN C (mg)
Breakfast	#1	430	22	357	4.3	2520	0.33	0.72	3.6	65
	#2	425	23	358	6.2	2300	0.54	1.03	5.4	61
	#3	400	19	346	4.7	2110	0.30	0.65	4.6	41
	#4	520	21	356	6.1	1575	0.72	1.02	7.1	78
	#5	345	35	361	4.9	7140	0.26	0.83	3.6	65
	#6	590	22	360	6.0	2320	0.81	0.96	7.7	137
	#7	440	20	387	4.3	4645	0.44	0.64	3.5	33
	#8	430	17	364	6.5	1720	0.80	1.06	7.3	23
	#9	365	31	341	4.0	445	0.34	0.66	3.7	62
	#10	425	14	374	6.2	1680	0.53	0.91	5.6	46

Diet Plan Number One
Nutritional Data

		ENERGY (cal)	PRO-TEIN (grams)	CAL-CIUM (mg)	IRON (mg)	VITAMIN A (IU)	THIAMIN (mg)	RIBO-FLAVIN (mg)	NIACIN (mg)	VITAMIN C (mg)
Lunch	#1	380	32	367	6.2	2010	0.31	0.50	6.2	106
	#2	415	37	314	6.2	4260	0.30	0.43	13.1	57
	#3	505	36	349	6.2	2060	0.39	0.51	7.0	89
	#4	555	40	371	6.2	4640	0.40	0.80	9.2	76
	#5	410	35	362	6.2	5360	0.31	0.79	6.1	38
	#6	450	22	318	6.3	3310	0.40	0.43	5.0	52
	#7	465	35	397	6.1	1670	0.31	0.81	5.1	27
	#8	420	35	457	6.3	2160	0.37	0.66	5.0	41
	#9	393	42	401	7.4	1050	0.31	0.88	5.5	99
	#10	390	22	412	7.1	2850	0.32	0.68	4.5	104

Diet Plan Number One
Nutritional Data

		PRO-TEIN (grams)	CAL-CIUM (mg)	IRON (mg)	VITAMIN A (IU)	THIAMIN (mg)	RIBO-FLAVIN (mg)	NIACIN (mg)	VITAMIN C (mg)
	ENERGY (cal)								
Dinner									
#1	360	31	274	8.3	10430	0.49	0.58	12.4	125
#2	430	29	310	8.4	5885	0.86	0.50	6.9	104
#3	490	34	290	8.0	22380	0.58	0.65	9.6	83
#4	410	39	508	8.1	21140	0.46	0.95	8.2	135
#5	396	43	404	8.2	4230	0.45	0.94	6.6	117
#6	515	31	285	9.1	3255	0.56	0.58	7.2	40
#7	415	33	278	8.3	14910	0.50	0.60	8.6	135
#8	367	33	284	9.7	5250	0.44	0.51	7.7	68
#9	445	34	381	8.2	31670	0.50	2.79	12.8	236
#10	270	27	383	15.0	4620	0.53	0.79	7.8	140

Diet Plan Number Two
Nutritional Data

	ENERGY (cal)	PRO-TEIN (grams)	CAL-CIUM (mg)	IRON (mg)	VITAMIN A (IU)	THIAMIN (mg)	RIBO-FLAVIN (mg)	NIACIN (mg)	VITAMIN C (mg)
Food Basket # 1	1002	74	900	18.0	62830	1.28	4.90	21.1	110
# 2	820	57	1027	18.3	5215	2.37	2.85	21.8	88
# 3	1070	60	1109	21.0	7690	1.13	1.41	13.0	66
# 4	865	61	986	21.0	10901	1.83	3.08	31.5	100
# 5	915	88	800	18.2	10310	1.00	2.69	17.5	108
# 6	1015	55	1015	21.3	5350	2.09	3.42	24.5	77
# 7	852	63	862	18.0	24918	1.03	1.96	15.5	232
# 8	990	60	852	18.0	12300	1.68	2.63	28.7	170
# 9	1240	79	836	18.7	5997	1.04	1.63	13.1	60
# 10	980	58	847	21.4	5025	2.02	3.19	29.9	65

17

EXERCISE AND
WEIGHT REDUCTION

DISMANTLING A MYTH

Mathematically, we know that there are three ways to tip the energy balance so that we may lose weight: we can diet, we can increase our activity, or we can institute a blend of the two.

And some form of low-calorie *dieting* is accepted by most people—and all real experts—as having value in weight reduction. By cutting down on eating, and thus ingesting fewer calories than we burn each day, we know that body weight will diminish. In fact, we've seen scientific proof of this in Chapter Fourteen.

But when the role of the second of the three methods is discussed, that of increased activity or more *exercise*, doubt is sometimes cast on its worth in an overall plan of weight reduction.

"Exercise does not consume enough calories" is the claim.

People will argue, for instance, that in order for a 160-pound woman to burn off one pound of body *fat* when walking at a moderately fast pace of 3.5 miles per hour (measurements indicate that walking at this speed burns 300 calories per hour), she would have to walk for 11.67 hours—during which time she would travel a distance of almost forty-one miles.* All this just to shed one pound of body weight through energy expenditure? Obviously impractical, these people would say; how much better it would be for her simply

---

*All other weight lost will be from perspiration—water weight only—and necessarily must be replaced by drinking liquids.

to excise some calories from her diet. Besides, they might go on, if she did all that work, her appetite would only increase to make up for the energy loss, and she would be right back where she started.

But the picture these people draw is one of too short range—and it is distorted. Their arithmetic is correct: exercise does require a lot of time to burn much in the way of calories. But our woman doesn't have to tackle that 11.67 hours of exercise all at once. She might split it up, walking one hour after dinner every day. If she did this, keeping food quantity the same, in twelve days she would lose over a pound of body fat; and if she were to maintain this schedule, she'd average a 2.5-pound drop a month—or over thirty pounds a year— or over sixty pounds in two years.

And suddenly the figures have become quite respectable, especially when stacked against the long span of time it takes for a person to grow excessively overweight.

And exercise can have an even more powerful effect than that. The typical American man expends about 3000 calories each day. In contrast, there are some elderly Swiss peasants who tend cattle in the Alps who average 5000 calories in expenditure daily. If our American man were to bring his energy output up to that of these Swiss while preserving his original eating habits, he would lose over a pound every two days, which is a high rate of weight loss.

Or, is it possible, as some detractors might say, that the additional exercise would only cause his appetite to increase in order to cover his new energy requirements—so that in the end he would not lose any weight?

No, not in this case.

At a certain level of energy expenditure the appestat and other survival apparatus assume control of body functions. Our man's appetite-energy regulating mechanisms would sense his great expansion of activity and would begin to prepare his system to meet these more severe demands by trimming excess weight from his body, now a liability, so that he could better endure under the new conditions. Gradually, the fat on his body would be disposed of, burned as fuel, and, as a consequence, body weight would decrease.

Once exercise has reached the range that allows the appestat and related mechanisms to operate properly, body weight is then controlled without conscious calorie counting and without a feeling of hunger. In weight reduction this is the one great advantage that exercise has over dieting.

But is the amount of exercise needed to sustain proper functioning of the appestat feasible in the context of today's living? Researchers at the Physical Fitness Laboratory of Wake Forest University conducted an exercise program for 16 sedentary middle-aged men, aged 40 to 56 years, that has helped to answer this question, while at the same time providing proof of the connection between exercise, appetite control, and weight reduction.

The subjects in this experiment were placed on a walking program in which they walked at the fast pace of 4.5 miles per hour for 40 minutes a day, four days a week, for twenty weeks. At the end of this time, though they had been permitted to eat as their appetites dictated, their body weights had gone down by an average of almost four pounds apiece.

The amount of weight they lost is significant, particularly when the free rein given to their appetites is considered. And when the gains in muscle, health, and fitness that accrued are also taken into account, the time they spent exercising each day is not unreasonable in length.

By dividing the 40 minutes of walking into two 20-minute periods, one morning and one evening four times a week, few people could not incorporate a program of this type into their daily schedules. And for the very busy there are more vigorous activities that require less time than walking for similar weight-appetite–regulation results.

GETTING STARTED

In this age of enlightenment most of us will admit that exercise is valuable. Besides the benefit of body-weight management, regular exercise will enhance physical fitness (strength, stamina, endurance), assist in the prevention of heart disease, on occasion influence the course of diabetes, many times cure insomnia, always upgrade physical appearance and mental self-image, and may very well be one of the keys to living a longer and happier life.

But despite knowledge of all this, we shun exercise. We're the victims of our inherited tendency toward laziness. And yet this instinct, passed down to us from our Stone Age ancestors, can be fought against and overcome.

First of all, just the recognition of where this desire to avoid activity comes from can help us negate its effect. When that subconscious voice whispers that we don't want to exercise, we'll know it originates from times long dead, that the information it is giving us is no longer valid, and that it's no longer imperative that we obey its instructions. With the smallest act of will power, then, we can safely ignore its promptings and begin a sensible exercise program.

Let's start.

The preliminary step is a physical examination by your doctor.

A small number of people are not medically ready to undertake an exercise program, and the unfortunate part is that they may not be aware that they have any problems. But these troubles, such as heart defects and respiratory ailments, often are unmasked after an exercise project has been entered into—sometimes to the detriment of health.

So get an okay to start from your physician.

Once you have it, you'll next want to select the form of exercise or activity you wish to engage in. There are several things here you'll need to take into consideration. First, you'll want to choose an exercise that expends a large number of calories for the time involved; also, you'll want it to be one that can be done over an extended period of time, and one that requires continuous deep breathing, since the oxygen inhaled is used in the oxidation of body fat for energy.

Many activities meet these criteria. Among the best are jogging, swimming, cycling, walking, stationary running, and rope skipping. Near to them in quality are basketball, handball, volleyball, squash, and tennis. But weight lifting, calisthenics, golf, and bowling, as generally practiced, have been shown by scientific measurement *not* to be vigorous and continuous enough for our purposes. Sometimes, however, these last activities can be modified to conform to the oxygen-requiring standard they must satisfy. For example, if you enjoy golf, by walking the fairways and carrying your clubs instead of driving a motorized cart, you can add a considerable number of calories to your energy expenditure over the nine or eighteen holes that you play. In this way, golf can be made to fall into line with the more potent of the energy-expending activities.

Nonetheless, whichever exercise you pick, engage in it at least four times a week, and preferably five.

But don't let any surge of ambition you might feel in the beginning carry you away so that you overwork yourself. Fatigue can cause injuries which will slow your progress or even bring it to an abrupt halt. Also, too much fatigue will kill your enthusiasm and you will find that you no longer look forward to exercising—with the result that you will quit.

To avoid these complications, plan a slow progression of workouts starting with easy-to-perform movements, or if you're starting on a walking or jogging program, commence with a slow pace and short times and distances. Then add to them in graduated steps. But every session should remain relatively easy to finish, especially during the first few months. So always end each exercising period before exhaustion sets in.

In any case, forcing is not productive. The human body contrives change in itself according to a phenomenon called the *overload principle*. Whenever the body is regularly forced to work a *little* harder than it normally does, it responds by increasing slightly its capacity to perform that activity—as a cushion or protection for itself, so that the next time it's called upon to complete that task, the effort will not be as taxing to the system.

Thus, with this built-in safeguard the body adapts itself to new and greater demands. The frames of marathon runners slowly trim down as they reach the distance of twenty-six miles; weight lifters and body builders steadily develop ever-larger muscles to cope with the increasingly heavier weights; swimmers discover that they can go an extra lap or that their times have come down. But the effect cannot be rushed. It progresses at a definite rate, so don't push too hard—it does no good.

And by not overworking, you won't dread each session, and in the end you'll achieve your goals of weight reduction and improved health more quickly.

TIPS ON EXERCISING

If you're the least bit undecided about which activity to pursue, let me make a suggestion: choose the exercise which requires the minimum amount of preparation and equipment, and which can be done at any time of day or night—walking.

You might embark on a walking program by initially strolling a half mile at a leisurely pace four or five times in the first week. (You can use the odometer of your car to measure distance on your route.)

With each succeeding week, still walking at your slow pace, you can add another half mile to your course. Do this for six weeks and you'll find that you are covering three miles—but you won't notice how far you've traveled. At the end of your stroll you'll feel relaxed and refreshed. Once you're walking this full route of three miles, you should gradually increase your speed until you're moving as rapidly as possible (but never exceeding limits of comfort). This is the rate of walking you should maintain from now on. It will insure adequate appetite-weight adjustment.

Besides its convenience, walking has a second advantage over the other methods of conditioning. It's inconspicuous. When you're doing it, nobody knows you're exercising.

You can carry a grocery bag with you, push the baby stroller, be accompanied by your spouse, drag the dog along on a leash, or just walk alone—all perfectly normal activities. Disguised, you won't be ridiculed or embarrassed as you condition your body. You'll be doing it secretly.

Still, you might feel too self-conscious to exercise in front of others, even if it's in the form of walking. But don't despair. There are two exercises which can be done behind closed doors that are effective for weight control and physical fitness. These movements are stationary running and rope skipping.

Stationary running, also known as running in place, is exactly what it sounds like. You lift your legs up and down as you do in jogging, but you stay in one spot. This exercise can be performed anywhere in your home, nobody sees you, and you avoid the rain, wind, and cold of the out-of-doors. To make it worthwhile, raise your feet eight inches or higher from the floor with each step. Rope skipping, the same as boxers do, is a little more challenging. It may take you a while to develop your skill. But no matter which you choose, over a period of two months or more lengthen the time you put in till you're exercising at least fifteen minutes a day, four or five days a week.

Should you feel that walking and the indoor activities are too tame, you might try jogging, swimming, or cycling.

Jogging is the best of all the aerobic (oxygen-requiring) exercises, burning the most calories for the time spent. It demands a good pair of soft-soled shoes and a minimum distance of one mile. Swimming ranks near jogging in effectiveness—suggested minimum distance to work up to: 600 yards. Cycling, on the other hand, is a very efficient form of movement; so your goal should be to ride at least five miles or more at a fast rate of speed.

Participating in sports in which other people are involved, like basketball, volleyball, and tennis, has its own unique problem. Dr. Jean Mayer of Harvard studied overweight adolescent girls taking part in such activities. Although the girls believed they were active throughout each period of play, Dr. Mayer discovered from a review of films that in reality they were motionless a good deal of the time. So when you're engaging in this type of activity, give some thought as to how much you're truly exercising, and try to keep moving as much as possible. It's to your benefit.

Here are some more hints you might find helpful.

At the end of each exercise session, taper off slowly, staying on your feet for five extra minutes to allow your body time to adjust itself down to its normal operating state. By walking around as you cool off, you'll prevent blood from pooling in your legs and thus reduce the possibility of fainting. Walking as a warm-up before exercise is also good.

As the weeks go by, the danger of resigning from your program because of monotony and boredom grows. You can combat this by varying the agenda: jogging over a different route, learning and perfecting a new stroke in swimming, or switching from the basketball court to the tennis court for a few weeks. Variety is one solution here.

A second way to beat the boredom problem is to exercise with other people. The conversation, camaraderie, and friendly rivalry will help to hold your interest. However, there are a couple of drawbacks to group activity. On occasion your fellows might not show up, and when they don't, you may not feel like exercising alone; or it may be impossible to go on without them—for instance, if a few sets of tennis had been planned. So pick reliable exercise partners.

Training at home, you might find a radio or record player suitable company.

Exercise does not always have to be a formalized program. You can enjoy many of the fruits of increased energy expenditure by simply altering your approach to everyday living. Spend an extra half-hour in the garden each evening; walk the kids to and from school rather than driving them in the car; use stairways instead of elevators; don't sit when you can stand; don't stand when you can move around.

Over the years this change in lifestyle, together with attention to diet, will pay handsome dividends in weight control, health, and fitness.

APPENDIX: NUTRITIVE VALUE
OF FOODS*

A glass of milk . . . a slice of cooked meat . . . an apple . . . a slice of bread—what food values does each contain? How much cooked meat will a pound of raw meat yield? How much protein is recommended a day for a healthy fourteen-year-old boy?

Ready answers to questions like these are helpful to homemakers who need quantitative information for the planning of nutritionally adequate diets, and to nutritionists, dietitians, and physicians.

The answers will be found in the tables.

EXPLANATION OF THE TABLES

About Table 1

Table 1 shows the food values in 615 foods commonly used in this country.

Foods listed.—Foods are grouped under the following main headings: milk; eggs; meat, poultry, and fish; dry beans and peas, nuts; vegetables; fruits; grain products; fats; sugars; and miscellaneous items.

*Home and Garden Bulletin No. 72, United States Department of Agriculture (Washington, D.C.: Superintendent of Documents, U.S. Goverment Printing Office, 1964; rev. 1964, 1970, 1971).

Most of the foods listed are in ready-to-eat form. Some are basic products widely used in food preparation, such as flour, fat, and cornmeal.

Weight in grams—rounded to the nearest whole gram—is shown for an approximate measure of each food as it is described; if inedible parts are included in the description, both measure and weight include these parts.

The approximate measure shown for each food is in cups, ounces, pounds, some other well-known unit, or a piece of certain size. Usually, the measure shown can be calculated to larger or smaller amounts by multiplying or dividing. Because the measures are approximate (some are rounded for convenient use), calculated nutritive values for larger quantities of some food items may be less representative than those calculated for smaller quantities.

The cup measure refers to the standard measuring cup of 8 fluid ounces or $\frac{1}{2}$ liquid pint. The ounce refers to $\frac{1}{16}$ of a pound avoirdupois, unless fluid ounce is indicated. The weight of a fluid ounce varies according to the food measures.

Factors in general use for converting from one measure to its equivalent in another measure include those shown below.

Equivalents by Volume
(All measurements level)

1 quart	= 4 cups
1 cup	= 8 fluid ounces
	= $\frac{1}{2}$ pint
	= 16 tablespoons
2 tablespoons	= 1 fluid ounce
1 tablespoon	= 3 teaspoons
1 pound regular butter or margarine	= 4 sticks
	= 2 cups
1 pound whipped butter or margarine	= 6 sticks
	= 2 8-ounce containers
	= 3 cups

EQUIVALENTS BY WEIGHT

1 pound (16 ounces)	= 453.6 grams
1 ounce	= 28.35 grams
3½ ounces	= 100 grams

Food values.—Values are shown for protein; fat; fatty acids; total carbohydrates; two minerals—calcium and iron; and five vitamins—vitamin A, thiamin, riboflavin, niacin, and ascorbic acid (vitamin C). Calories are shown in the column headed "Food energy." The calorie is the unit of measure for the energy furnished the body by protein, fat, and carbohydrate.

These values can be used as the basis for comparing kinds and amounts of nutrients in different foods. For some foods, the values can be used in comparing different forms of the same food.

Water content is also shown in the table because the percentage of moisture present is needed for identification and comparison of many food items.

The values for food energy (calories) and nutrients shown in Table 1 are the amounts present in the edible part of the item, that is, in only that portion of the weight of the item customarily eaten—corn without cob, meat without bone, potatoes without skin, European-type grapes without seeds. If additional parts are eaten—the skin of the potato, for example—amounts of some nutrients obtained will be somewhat greater than those shown.

For many of the prepared items, values have been calculated from the ingredients in typical recipes. Examples of such items are: Biscuits, corn muffins, oyster stew, macaroni and cheese, custard, and a number of other dessert-type items.

For toast and for vegetables, values are without fat added, either during preparation or at the table. Values for the thiamin content of toast are about 20 percent lower than for fresh bread; it was impossible to show this loss adequately because of the small amount of thiamin present in a slice of bread. Some destruction of vitamins in vegetables, especially of ascorbic acid, may occur when foods are cut or shredded.

Such losses are variable, and no deduction for these losses has been made.

For meat, values are for meat as cooked, drained, and without drippings. For many cuts, two sets of values are shown: Meat including the fat, and meat from which the fat has been trimmed off in the kitchen or on the plate.

A variety of manufactured items, such as some of the milk products, ready-to-eat breakfast cereals, imitation cream products, fruit drinks, and various mixes are included in Table 1. Frequently these foods are fortified with one or more nutrients. If nutrients are added, this information is on the label. Values shown in this bulletin for these foods are usually based on products from several manufacturers and may differ somewhat from the values provided by any one source.

Yield of Cooked Meat

Meat undergoes certain losses from the time it is purchased to the time it is ready to serve. Among these losses are those that occur through evaporation of moisture, loss of fat in the drippings, and discard of bone and various trimming.

See the relationships between weights of raw meat as purchased and yield of cooked meat. The approximate weight of cooked, drained meat that usually can be expected from a pound of raw meat as purchased in several cuts is shown. Yield is given as ounces of—

Cooked meat with bone and fat
Cooked lean and fat
Cooked lean only

Among the factors that influence the yield of meat is the proportion of fat and lean in the piece. Many cuts have a layer of fat extending all or part way around. The thickness of this fat varies because practices in cutting and trimming meat for retail distribution differ widely. The data on yield of meat as well as those on nutritive value in Table 1, apply to cuts trimmed so that the outer layer of fat is not more than $\frac{1}{2}$ inch in thickness. Deposits of fat within a cut may be extensive and usually are not affected by retail trimming although they may be discarded at the table.

About Table 2

Table 2 shows Recommended Daily Dietary Allowances for calories and for several nutrients essential for maintenance of good nutrition in healthy, normally active persons in this country. This table is an abbreviated version which has been adapted from more extensive material published in 1968 by the Food and Nutrition Board, National Academy of Sciences–National Research Council.

Additional nutrients for which the Food and Nutrition Board published Recommended Daily Dietary Allowances are: The B-vitamins—vitamins B6, B12, and folacin, vitamins D and E, phosphorus, magnesium, and iodine.

Data for these nutrients are not shown in Table 1 of this appendix, and the allowances for them have been omitted from Table 2. However, foods which are of special value in supplying these eight nutrients (either because they are high in the nutrient or because quantities generally eaten supply relatively large amounts) are listed.

The allowance of 18 milligrams of iron per day recommended for girls and women is almost impossible to obtain through ordinary foods; iron supplementation is often required. Many foods, for example, breakfast cereals, are being fortified with iron at increasingly higher levels to meet this allowance for girls and women.

More detailed information about the Recommended Daily Allowances may be obtained from the publication from which Table 2 is adapted (see source note at the bottom of table.).

VITAMIN B6
Bananas
Whole-grain cereals
Chicken
Dry legumes
Egg yolk
Most dark-green leafy
vegetables
Most fish and shellfish
Muscle meats, liver,
and kidney
Peanuts, walnuts, filberts,
peanut butter
Potatoes and sweet potatoes
Prunes and raisins
Yeast

FOLACIN
Liver
Dark-green vegetables
Dry beans
Peanuts, walnuts, filberts
Lentils

Meat
Milk
Most cheeses
Most fish
Shellfish
Whole egg and egg yolk

VITAMIN E
Vegetable oils
Margarine
Salad dressing
Whole-grain cereals
Peanuts

VITAMIN D
Vitamin D milks
Egg yolk
Salt-water fish
Liver

MAGNESIUM
Bananas
Whole-grain cereals
Dry beans
Milk
Most dark-green leafy vegetables
Nuts
Peanuts, peanut butter

PHOSPHORUS
Whole-grain cereals
Cheese
Dry beans
Eggs
Meat
Milk
Peanuts, peanut butter

VITAMIN B12 (*present
in foods of animal
origin only*)
Kidney
Liver

IODINE
Iodized salt
Seafood

Niacin and Niacin Equivalent

Niacin, for which values are given in Table 1, is a less inclusive term than niacin equivalent used in Table 2. Nearly all foods contain some tryptophan, an amino acid found in protein, which the body can convert to niacin. Niacin equivalent is the composite of the niacin already in the food and that which may be formed from tryptophan. Among the better sources of trypotophan are milk, meats, eggs, legumes, and nuts.

In the United States, the average diet contains a generous amount of protein, and provides enough tryptophan to increase the niacin value calculated from Table 1 by about a third.

More Information from USDA

A number of other publications of the Agricultural Research Service, U.S. Department of Agriculture, give helpful information about nutrients and where they are found in foods.

Single copies of the following bulletins are free from the Office of Information, U.S. Department of Agriculture, Washington, D.C. 20250. Send your request on a post card and include your zip code.

Family Fare: A Guide to Good Nutrition ....G 1
Food and Your Weight ....G 74
Conserving the Nutritive Values in Foods..........G 90
Calories and Weight: The USDA Pocket Guide ......G 153

Those interested in learning more about tables of nutritive values can order Yearbook Separate No. 3666, "Nutritive Values of Foods and Use of Tables Listing Them." This reprint from the 1969 Yearbook of Agriculture, "Food for Us All," is also available free from the Office of Information, U.S. Department of Agriculture at the above address.

For a more highly technical publication with data on a much more extensive list of foods, see Agriculture Handbook No. 8, "Composition of Foods . . . raw, processed, prepared." In this handbook data are presented for the nutrients in 100 grams of edible portion and one pound of food as purchased. The handbook is for sale by the Superintendent of Documents, U.S. Government Printing Office, Washington, D.C. 20402.

TABLE 1.—NUTRITIVE VALUES OF THE

	Food, approximate measure, and weight (in grams)		Water	Food energy	Pro-tein	Fat
	MILK, CHEESE, CREAM, IMITATION CREAM; RELATED PRODUCTS					
		Grams	*Per-cent*	*Calo-ries*	*Grams*	*Grams*
	Milk:					
	Fluid:					
1	Whole, 3.5% fat_____ 1 cup_____	244	87	160	9	9
2	Nonfat (skim)_____ 1 cup_____	245	90	90	9	Trace
3	Partly skimmed, 2% 1 cup_____ nonfat milk solids added.	246	87	145	10	5
	Canned, concentrated, undiluted:					
4	Evaporated, un- 1 cup_____ sweetened.	252	74	345	18	20
5	Condensed, sweet- 1 cup_____ ened.	306	27	980	25	27
	Dry, nonfat instant:					
6	Low-density (1⅓ 1 cup_____ cups needed for re-constitution to 1 qt.).	68	4	245	24	Trace
7	High-density (⅞ cup 1 cup_____ needed for recon-stitution to 1 qt.).	104	4	375	37	1
	Buttermilk:					
8	Fluid, cultured, made 1 cup_____ from skim milk.	245	90	90	9	Trace
9	Dried, packaged_____ 1 cup_____	120	3	465	41	6
	Cheese:					
	Natural:					
	Blue or Roquefort type:					
10	Ounce_____ 1 oz._____	28	40	105	6	9
11	Cubic inch_____ 1 cu. in._____	17	40	65	4	5

(Dashes in the columns for nutrients show that no suitable value could be found although there is reason to believe that a measurable amount of the nutrient may be present)

EDIBLE PART OF FOODS

Fatty acids			Carbo-hy-drate	Cal-cium	Iron	Vita-min A value	Thia-min	Ribo-flavin	Niacin	Ascor-bic acid
Satu-rated (total)	Unsaturated									
	Oleic	Lin-oleic								
Grams	Grams	Grams	Grams	Milli-grams	Milli-grams	Inter-national units	Milli-grams	Milli-grams	Milli-grams	Milli-grams
5	3	Trace	12	288	0.1	350	0.07	0.41	0.2	2
------	------	------	12	296	.1	10	.09	.44	.2	2
3	2	Trace	15	352	.1	200	.10	.52	.2	2
11	7	1	24	635	.3	810	.10	.86	.5	3
15	9	1	166	802	.3	1,100	.24	1.16	.6	3
------	------	------	35	879	.4	[1]20	.24	1.21	.6	5
------	------	------	54	1,345	.6	[1]30	.36	1.85	.9	7
------	------	------	12	296	.1	10	.10	.44	.2	2
3	2	Trace	60	1,498	.7	260	.31	2.06	1.1	------
5	3	Trace	1	89	.1	350	.01	.17	.3	0
3	2	Trace	Trace	54	.1	210	.01	.11	.2	0

[1]Value applies to unfortified product; value for fortified low-density product would be 1500 I.U. and the fortified high-density product would be 2290 I.U.

TABLE 1.—NUTRITIVE VALUES OF THE

	Food, approximate measure, and weight (in grams)			Water	Food energy	Pro-tein	Fat
	MILK, CHEESE, CREAM, IMITATION CREAM; RELATED PRODUCTS—Con.						
	Cheese—Continued						
	Natural—Continued		*Grams*	*Per-cent*	*Calo-ries*	*Grams*	*Grams*
12	Camembert, pack-aged in 4-oz. pkg. with 3 wedges per pkg.	1 wedge	38	52	115	7	9
	Cheddar:						
13	Ounce	1 oz.	28	37	115	7	9
14	Cubic inch	1 cu. in.	17	37	70	4	6
	Cottage, large or small curd:						
	Creamed:						
15	Package of 12-oz., net wt.	1 pkg.	340	78	360	46	14
16	Cup, curd pressed down.	1 cup	245	78	260	33	10
	Uncreamed:						
17	Package of 12-oz., net wt.	1 pkg.	340	79	290	58	1
18	Cup, curd pressed down.	1 cup	200	79	170	34	1
	Cream:						
19	Package of 8-oz., net wt.	1 pkg.	227	51	850	18	86
20	Package of 3-oz., net wt.	1 pkg.	85	51	320	7	32
21	Cubic inch	1 cu. in.	16	51	60	1	6
	Parmesan, grated:						
22	Cup, pressed down	1 cup	140	17	655	60	43
23	Tablespoon	1 tbsp.	5	17	25	2	2
24	Ounce	1 oz.	28	17	130	12	9
	Swiss:						
25	Ounce	1 oz.	28	39	105	8	8
26	Cubic inch	1 cu. in.	15	39	55	4	4

Fatty acids			Carbo-hy-drate	Cal-cium	Iron	Vita-min A value	Thia-min	Ribo-flavin	Niacin	Ascor-bic acid
Satu-rated (total)	Unsaturated									
	Oleic	Lin-oleic								
Grams	*Grams*	*Grams*	*Grams*	*Milli-grams*	*Milli-grams*	*Inter-national units*	*Milli-grams*	*Milli-grams*	*Milli-grams*	*Milli-grams*
5	3	Trace	1	40	0.2	380	0.02	0.29	0.3	0
5	3	Trace	1	213	.3	370	.01	.13	Trace	0
3	2	Trace	Trace	129	.2	230	.01	.08	Trace	0
8	5	Trace	10	320	1.0	580	.10	.85	.3	0
6	3	Trace	7	230	.7	420	.07	.61	.2	0
1	Trace	Trace	9	306	1.4	30	.10	.95	.3	0
Trace	Trace	Trace	5	180	.8	20	.06	.56	.2	0
48	28	3	5	141	.5	3,500	.05	.54	.2	0
18	11	1	2	53	.2	1,310	.02	.20	.1	0
3	2	Trace	Trace	10	Trace	250	Trace	.04	Trace	0
24	14	1	5	1,893	.7	1,760	.03	1.22	.3	0
1	Trace	Trace	Trace	68	Trace	60	Trace	.04	Trace	0
5	3	Trace	1	383	.1	360	.01	.25	.1	0
4	3	Trace	1	262	.3	320	Trace	.11	Trace	0
2	1	Trace	Trace	139	.1	170	Trace	.06	Trace	0

TABLE 1.—NUTRITIVE VALUES OF THE

	Food, approximate measure, and weight (in grams)			Water	Food energy	Pro-tein	Fat
	MILK, CHEESE, CREAM, IMITATION CREAM; RELATED PRODUCTS—Con.						
	Cheese—Continued		Grams	Per-cent	Calo-ries	Grams	Grams
	Pasteurized processed cheese:						
	American:						
27	Ounce_____ 1 oz._____		28	40	105	7	9
28	Cubic inch_____ 1 cu. in._____		18	40	65	4	5
	Swiss:						
29	Ounce_____ 1 oz._____		28	40	100	8	8
30	Cubic inch_____ 1 cu. in._____		18	40	65	5	5
	Pasteurized process cheese food, American:						
31	Tablespoon_____ 1 tbsp._____		14	43	45	3	3
32	Cubic inch_____ 1 cu. in._____		18	43	60	4	4
33	Pasteurized process 1 oz._____ cheese spread, American.		28	49	80	5	6
	Cream:						
34	Half-and-half (cream 1 cup_____ and milk).		242	80	325	8	28
35	1 tbsp._____		15	80	20	1	2
36	Light, coffee or table___ 1 cup_____		240	72	505	7	49
37	1 tbsp._____		15	72	30	1	3
38	Sour_____ 1 cup_____		230	72	485	7	47
39	1 tbsp._____		12	72	25	Trace	2
40	Whipped topping 1 cup_____ (pressurized).		60	62	155	2	14
41	1 tbsp._____		3	62	10	Trace	1
	Whipping, unwhipped (volume about double when whipped):						
42	Light_____ 1 cup_____		239	62	715	6	75
43	1 tbsp._____		15	62	45	Trace	5
44	Heavy_____ 1 cup_____		238	57	840	5	90
45	1 tbsp._____		15	57	55	Trace	6

EDIBLE PART OF FOODS *(continued)*

Fatty acids			Carbo-hydrate	Cal-cium	Iron	Vita-min A value	Thia-min	Ribo-flavin	Niacin	Ascor-bic acid
Satu-rated (total)	Unsaturated									
	Oleic	Lin-oleic								
Grams	*Grams*	*Grams*	*Grams*	*Milli-grams*	*Milli-grams*	*Inter-national units*	*Milli-grams*	*Milli-grams*	*Milli-grams*	*Milli-grams*
5	3	Trace	1	198	.3	350	.01	.12	Trace	0
3	2	Trace	Trace	122	.2	210	Trace	.07	Trace	0
4	3	Trace	1	251	.3	310	Trace	.11	Trace	0
3	2	Trace	Trace	159	.2	200	Trace	.07	Trace	0
2	1	Trace	1	80	.1	140	Trace	.08	Trace	0
2	1	Trace	1	100	.1	170	Trace	.10	Trace	0
3	2	Trace	2	160	.2	250	Trace	.15	Trace	0
15	9	1	11	261	.1	1,160	.07	.39	.1	2
1	1	Trace	1	16	Trace	70	Trace	.02	Trace	Trace
27	16	1	10	245	.1	2,020	.07	.36	.1	2
2	1	Trace	1	15	Trace	130	Trace	.02	Trace	Trace
26	16	1	10	235	.1	1,930	.07	.35	.1	2
1	1	Trace	1	12	Trace	100	Trace	.02	Trace	Trace
8	5	Trace	6	67	------	570	------	.04	------	------
Trace	Trace	Trace	Trace	3	------	30	------	Trace	------	------
41	25	2	9	203	.1	3,060	.05	.29	.1	2
3	2	Trace	1	13	Trace	190	Trace	.02	Trace	Trace
50	30	3	7	179	.1	3,670	.05	.26	.1	2
3	2	Trace	1	11	Trace	230	Trace	.02	Trace	Trace

TABLE 1.—NUTRITIVE VALUES OF THE

	Food, approximate measure, and weight (in grams)		Water	Food energy	Pro-tein	Fat
	MILK, CHEESE, CREAM, IMITATION CREAM; RELATED PRODUCTS—Con.	*Grams*	*Per-cent*	*Calo-ries*	*Grams*	*Grams*
	Imitation cream products (made with vegetable fat):					
	Creamers:					
46	Powdered_____ 1 cup_____	94	2	505	4	33
47	1 tsp._____	2	2	10	Trace	1
48	Liquid (frozen)_____ 1 cup_____	245	77	345	3	27
49	1 tbsp._____	15	77	20	Trace	2
50	Sour dressing (imita- 1 cup_____ tion sour cream) made with nonfat dry milk.	235	72	440	9	38
51	1 tbsp._____	12	72	20	Trace	2
	Whipped topping:					
52	Pressurized_____ 1 cup_____	70	61	190	1	17
53	1 tbsp._____	4	61	10	Trace	1
54	Frozen_____ 1 cup_____	75	52	230	1	20
55	1 tbsp._____	4	52	10	Trace	1
56	Powdered, made with 1 cup_____ whole milk.	75	58	175	3	12
57	1 tbsp._____	4	58	10	Trace	1
	Milk beverages:					
58	Cocoa, homemade_____ 1 cup_____	250	79	245	10	12
59	Chocolate-flavored 1 cup_____ drink made with skim milk and 2% added butterfat.	250	83	190	8	6
	Malted milk:					
60	Dry powder, approx. 1 oz._____ 3 heaping tea-spoons per ounce.	28	3	115	4	2
61	Beverage_____ 1 cup_____	235	78	245	11	10

[2]Contributed largely from beta-carotene used for coloring.

EDIBLE PART OF FOODS *(continued)*

Fatty acids			Carbo-hy-drate	Cal-cium	Iron	Vita-min A value	Thia-min	Ribo-flavin	Niacin	Ascor-bic acid
Satu-rated (total)	Unsaturated									
	Oleic	Lin-oleic								
Grams	Grams	Grams	Grams	Milli-grams	Milli-grams	Inter-national units	Milli-grams	Milli-grams	Milli-grams	Milli-grams
31	1	0	52	21	.6	[2]200	------	------	Trace	------
Trace	Trace	0	1	1	Trace	[2]Trace	------	------	------	------
25	1	0	25	29	------	[2]100	0	0	------	------
1	Trace	0	2	2	------	[2]10	0	0	------	------
35	1	Trace	17	277	.1	10	.07	.38	.2	1
2	Trace	Trace	1	14	Trace	Trace	Trace	Trace	Trace	Trace
15	1	0	9	5	------	[2]340	------	0	------	------
1	Trace	0	Trace	Trace	------	[2]20	------	0	------	------
18	Trace	0	15	5	------	[2]560	------	0	------	------
1	Trace	0	1	Trace	------	[2]30	------	0	------	------
10	1	Trace	15	62	Trace	[2]330	.02	.08	.1	Trace
1	Trace	Trace	1	3	Trace	[2]20	Trace	Trace	Trace	Trace
7	4	Trace	27	295	1.0	400	.10	.45	.5	3
3	2	Trace	27	270	.5	210	.10	.40	.3	3
------	------	------	20	82	.6	290	.09	.15	.1	0
------	------	------	28	317	.7	590	.14	.49	.2	2

TABLE 1.—NUTRITIVE VALUES OF THE

	Food, approximate measure, and weight (in grams)			Water	Food energy	Protein	Fat
	MILK, CHEESE, CREAM, IMITATION CREAM; RELATED PRODUCTS—Con.						
			Grams	*Percent*	*Calories*	*Grams*	*Grams*
	Milk desserts:						
62	Custard, baked_____	1 cup_____	265	77	305	14	15
	Ice cream:						
63	Regular (approx. 10% fat).	½ gal._____	1,064	63	2,055	48	113
64		1 cup_____	133	63	255	6	14
65		3 fl. oz. cup__	50	63	95	2	5
66	Rich (approx. 16% fat).	½ gal._____	1,188	63	2,635	31	191
67		1 cup_____	148	63	330	4	24
	Ice milk:						
68	Hardened_____	½ gal._____	1,048	67	1,595	50	53
69		1 cup_____	131	67	200	6	7
70	Soft-serve_____	1 cup_____	175	67	265	8	9
	Yoghurt:						
71	Made from partially skimmed milk.	1 cup_____	245	89	125	8	4
72	Made from whole milk_	1 cup_____	245	88	150	7	8
	EGGS						
	Eggs, large, 24 ounces per dozen:						
	Raw or cooked in shell or with nothing added:						
73	Whole, without shell_	1 egg_____	50	74	80	6	6
74	White of egg_____	1 white_____	33	88	15	4	Trace
75	Yolk of egg_____	1 yolk_____	17	51	60	3	5
76	Scrambled with milk and fat.	1 egg_____	64	72	110	7	8

EDIBLE PART OF FOODS *(continued)*

Fatty acids			Carbo-hy-drate	Cal-cium	Iron	Vita-min A value	Thia-min	Ribo-flavin	Niacin	Ascor-bic acid
Satu-rated (total)	Unsaturated									
	Oleic	Lin-oleic								
Grams	Grams	Grams	Grams	Milli-grams	Milli-grams	Inter-national units	Milli-grams	Milli-grams	Milli-grams	Milli-grams
7	5	1	29	297	1.1	930	.11	.50	.3	1
62	37	3	221	1,553	.5	4,680	.43	2.23	1.1	11
8	5	Trace	28	194	.1	590	.05	.28	.1	1
3	2	Trace	10	73	Trace	220	.02	.11	.1	1
105	63	6	214	927	.2	7,840	.24	1.31	1.2	12
13	8	1	27	115	Trace	980	.03	.16	.1	1
29	17	2	235	1,635	1.0	2,200	.52	2.31	1.0	10
4	2	Trace	29	204	.1	280	.07	.29	.1	1
5	3	Trace	39	273	.2	370	.09	.39	.2	2
2	1	Trace	13	294	.1	170	.10	.44	.2	2
5	3	Trace	12	272	.1	340	.07	.39	.2	2
2	3	Trace	Trace	27	1.1	590	.05	.15	Trace	0
-----	-----	-----	Trace	3	Trace	0	Trace	.09	Trace	0
2	2	Trace	Trace	24	.9	580	.04	.07	Trace	0
3	3	Trace	1	51	1.1	690	.05	.18	Trace	0

TABLE 1.—NUTRITIVE VALUES OF THE

	Food, approximate measure, and weight (in grams)	Water	Food energy	Pro-tein	Fat
	MEAT, POULTRY, FISH, SHELLFISH; RELATED PRODUCTS	*Per-cent*	*Calo-ries*	*Grams*	*Grams*
		Grams			
77	Bacon, (20 slices per lb. 2 slices_____ raw), broiled or fried, crisp.	15	8	90	5	8
	Beef,[3] cooked:					
	Cuts braised, simmered, or pot-roasted:					
78	Lean and fat_____ 3 ounces_____	85	53	245	23	16
79	Lean only_____ 2.5 ounces___	72	62	140	22	5
	Hamburger (ground beef), broiled:					
80	Lean_____ 3 ounces_____	85	60	185	23	10
81	Regular_____ 3 ounces_____	85	54	245	21	17
	Roast, oven-cooked, no liquid added:					
	Relatively fat, such as rib:					
82	Lean and fat_____ 3 ounces_____	85	40	375	17	34
83	Lean only_____ 1.8 ounces___	51	57	125	14	7
	Relatively lean, such as heel of round:					
84	Lean and fat_____ 3 ounces_____	85	62	165	25	7
85	Lean only_____ 2.7 ounces___	78	65	125	24	3
	Steak, broiled:					
	Relatively, fat, such as sirloin:					
86	Lean and fat_____ 3 ounces_____	85	44	330	20	27
87	Lean only_____ 2.0 ounces___	56	59	115	18	4
	Relatively, lean, such as round:					
88	Lean and fat_____ 3 ounces_____	85	55	220	24	13
89	Lean only_____ 2.4 ounces___	68	61	130	21	4
	Beef, canned:					
90	Corned beef_____ 3 ounces_____	85	59	185	22	10
91	Corned beef hash_____ 3 ounces_____	85	67	155	7	10
92	Beef, dried or chipped____ 2 ounces_____	57	48	115	19	4
93	Beef and vegetable stew__ 1 cup_____	235	82	210	15	10

[3]Outer layer of fat on the cut was removed to within approximately ½-inch of the lean. Deposits of fat within the cut were not removed.

EDIBLE PART OF FOODS (*continued*)

Fatty acids			Carbo-hydrate	Cal-cium	Iron	Vita-min A value	Thia-min	Ribo-flavin	Niacin	Ascorbic acid
Satu-rated (total)	Unsaturated									
	Oleic	Lin-oleic								
Grams	Grams	Grams	Grams	Milli-grams	Milli-grams	Inter-national units	Milli-grams	Milli-grams	Milli-grams	Milli-grams
3	4	1	1	2	.5	0	.08	.05	.8	------
8	7	Trace	0	10	2.9	30	.04	.18	3.5	------
2	2	Trace	0	10	2.7	10	.04	.16	3.3	------
5	4	Trace	0	10	3.0	20	.08	.20	5.1	------
8	8	Trace	0	9	2.7	30	.07	.18	4.6	------
16	15	1	0	8	2.2	70	.05	.13	3.1	------
3	3	Trace	0	6	1.8	10	.04	.11	2.6	------
3	3	Trace	0	11	3.2	10	.06	.19	4.5	------
1	1	Trace	0	10	3.0	Trace	.06	.18	4.3	------
13	12	1	0	9	2.5	50	.05	.16	4.0	------
2	2	Trace	0	7	2.2	10	.05	.14	3.6	------
6	6	Trace	0	10	3.0	20	.07	.19	4.8	------
2	2	Trace	0	9	2.5	10	.06	.16	4.1	------
5	4	Trace	0	17	3.7	20	.01	.20	2.9	------
5	4	Trace	9	11	1.7	-------	.01	.08	1.8	------
2	2	Trace	0	11	2.9	-------	.04	.18	2.2	------
5	4	Trace	15	28	2.8	2,310	.13	.17	4.4	15

TABLE 1.—NUTRITIVE VALUES OF THE

	Food, approximate measure, and weight (in grams)			Water	Food energy	Pro-tein	Fat
	MEAT, POULTRY, FISH, SHELLFISH; RELATED PRODUCTS—Continued			*Per-cent*	*Calo-ries*	*Grams*	*Grams*
			Grams				
94	Beef potpie, baked, 4¼-inch diam., weight before baking about 8 ounces.	1 pie_____	227	55	560	23	33
	Chicken, cooked:						
95	Flesh only, broiled_____	3 ounces_____	85	71	115	20	3
	Breast, fried, ½ breast:						
96	With bone_____	3.3 ounces___	94	58	155	25	5
97	Flesh and skin only__	2.7 ounces___	76	58	155	25	5
	Drumstick, fried:						
98	With bone_____	2.1 ounces___	59	55	90	12	4
99	Flesh and skin only__	1.3 ounces___	38	55	90	12	4
100	Chicken, canned, boneless	3 ounces___	85	65	170	18	10
101	Chicken potpie, baked 4¼-inch diam., weight before baking about 8 ounces.	1 pie_____	227	57	535	23	31
	Chili con carne, canned:						
102	With beans_____	1 cup_____	250	72	335	19	15
103	Without beans_____	1 cup_____	255	67	510	26	38
104	Heart, beef, lean, braised_	3 ounces_____	85	61	160	27	5
	Lamb,[3] cooked:						
105	Chop, thick, with bone, broiled.	1 chop, 4.8 ounces.	137	47	400	25	33
106	Lean and fat_____	4.0 ounces___	112	47	400	25	33
107	Lean only_____	2.6 ounces___	74	62	140	21	6
	Leg, roasted:						
108	Lean and fat_____	3 ounces_____	85	54	235	22	16
109	Lean only_____	2.5 ounces___	71	62	130	20	5
	Shoulder, roasted:						
110	Lean and fat_____	3 ounces_____	85	50	285	18	23
111	Lean only_____	2.3 ounces___	64	61	130	17	6

EDIBLE PART OF FOODS (*continued*)

Fatty acids			Carbo-hydrate	Calcium	Iron	Vitamin A value	Thiamin	Riboflavin	Niacin	Ascorbic acid
Saturated (total)	Unsaturated									
	Oleic	Linoleic								
Grams	*Grams*	*Grams*	*Grams*	*Milligrams*	*Milligrams*	*International units*	*Milligrams*	*Milligrams*	*Milligrams*	*Milligrams*
9	20	2	43	32	4.1	1,860	0.25	0.27	4.5	7
1	1	1	0	8	1.4	80	.05	.16	7.4	------
1	2	1	1	9	1.3	70	.04	.17	11.2	------
1	2	1	1	9	1.3	70	.04	.17	11.2	------
1	2	1	Trace	6	.9	50	.03	.15	2.7	------
1	2	1	Trace	6	.9	50	.03	.15	2.7	------
3	4	2	0	18	1.3	200	.03	.11	3.7	3
10	15	3	42	68	3.0	3,020	.25	.26	4.1	5
7	7	Trace	30	80	4.2	150	.08	.18	3.2	------
18	17	1	15	97	3.6	380	.05	.31	5.6	------
------	------	------	1	5	5.0	20	.21	1.04	6.5	1
18	12	1	0	10	1.5	------	.14	.25	5.6	------
18	12	1	0	10	1.5	------	.14	.25	5.6	------
3	2	Trace	0	9	1.5	------	.11	.20	4.5	------
9	6	Trace	0	9	1.4	------	.13	.23	4.7	------
3	2	Trace	0	9	1.4	------	.12	.21	4.4	------
13	8	1	0	9	1.0	------	.11	.20	4.0	------
3	2	Trace	0	8	1.0	------	.10	.18	3.7	------

TABLE 1.—NUTRITIVE VALUES OF THE

	Food, approximate measure, and weight (in grams)		Grams	Water	Food energy	Pro-tein	Fat
	MEAT, POULTRY, FISH, SHELLFISH; RELATED PRODUCTS—Continued			*Per-cent*	*Calo-ries*	*Grams*	*Grams*
112	Liver, beef, fried_____	2 ounces_____	57	57	130	15	6
	Pork, cured, cooked:						
113	Ham, light cure, lean and fat, roasted.	3 ounces_____	85	54	245	18	19
	Luncheon meat:						
114	Boiled ham, sliced___	2 ounces_____	57	59	135	11	10
115	Canned, spiced or unspiced.	2 ounces_____	57	55	165	8	14
	Pork, fresh,[3] cooked:						
116	Chop, thick, with bone_	1 chop, 3.5 ounces.	98	42	260	16	21
117	Lean and fat_____	2.3 ounces___	66	42	260	16	21
118	Lean only_____	1.7 ounces___	48	53	130	15	7
	Roast, oven-cooked, no liquid added:						
119	Lean and fat_____	3 ounces_____	85	46	310	21	24
120	Lean only_____	2.4 ounces___	68	55	175	20	10
	Cuts, simmered:						
121	Lean and fat_____	3 ounces_____	85	46	320	20	26
122	Lean only_____	2.2 ounces___	63	60	135	18	6
	Sausage:						
123	Bologna, slice, 3-in. diam. by ⅛ inch.	2 slices_____	26	56	80	3	7
124	Braunschweiger, slice 2-in. diam. by ¼ inch.	2 slices_____	20	53	65	3	5
125	Deviled ham, canned___	1 tbsp._____	13	51	45	2	4
126	Frankfurter, heated (8 per lb. purchased pkg.).	1 frank_____	56	57	170	7	15
127	Pork links, cooked (16 links per lb. raw).	2 links_____	26	35	125	5	11

[3]Outer layer of fat on the cut was removed to within approximately ½-inch of the lean. Deposits of fat within the cut were not removed.

EDIBLE PART OF FOODS (continued)

Fatty acids			Carbo-hydrate	Cal-cium	Iron	Vita-min A value	Thia-min	Ribo-flavin	Niacin	Ascor-bic acid
Satu-rated (total)	Unsaturated									
	Oleic	Lin-oleic								
Grams	Grams	Grams	Grams	Milli-grams	Milli-grams	Inter-national units	Milli-grams	Milli-grams	Milli-grams	Milli-grams
------	------	------	3	6	5.0	30,280	.15	2.37	9.4	15
7	8	2	0	8	2.2	0	.40	.16	3.1	------
4	4	1	0	6	1.6	0	.25	.09	1.5	------
5	6	1	1	5	1.2	0	.18	.12	1.6	------
8	9	2	0	8	2.2	0	.63	.18	3.8	------
8	9	2	0	8	2.2	0	.63	.18	3.8	------
2	3	1	0	7	1.9	0	.54	.16	3.3	------
9	10	2	0	9	2.7	0	.78	.22	4.7	------
3	4	1	0	9	2.6	0	.73	.21	4.4	------
9	11	2	0	8	2.5	0	.46	.21	4.1	------
2	3	1	0	8	2.3	0	.42	.19	3.7	------
------	------	------	Trace	2	.5	-------	.04	.06	.7	------
------	------	------	Trace	2	1.2	1,310	.03	.29	1.6	------
2	2	Trace	0	1	.3	-------	.02	.01	.2	------
------	------	------	1	3	.8	-------	.08	.11	1.4	------
4	5	1	Trace	2	.6	0	.21	.09	1.0	------

TABLE 1.—NUTRITIVE VALUES OF THE

Food, approximate measure, and weight (in grams)			Water	Food energy	Pro-tein	Fat

MEAT, POULTRY, FISH, SHELLFISH; RELATED PRODUCTS—Continued

			Grams	*Per-cent*	*Calo-ries*	*Grams*	*Grams*
	Sausage—Continued						
128	Salami, dry type_____	1 oz._____	28	30	130	7	11
129	Salami, cooked_____	1 oz._____	28	51	90	5	7
130	Vienna, canned (7 sausages per 5-oz. can).	1 sausage____	16	63	40	2	3
	Veal, medium fat, cooked, bone removed:						
131	Cutlet_____	3 oz._____	85	60	185	23	9
132	Roast_____	3 oz._____	85	55	230	23	14
	Fish and shellfish:						
133	Bluefish, baked with table fat.	3 oz._____	85	68	135	22	4
	Clams:						
134	Raw, meat only_____	3 oz._____	85	82	65	11	1
135	Canned, solids and liquid.	3 oz._____	85	86	45	7	1
136	Crabmeat, canned_____	3 oz._____	85	77	85	15	2
137	Fish sticks, breaded, cooked, frozen; stick 3¾ by 1 by ½ inch.	10 sticks or 8 oz. pkg.	227	66	400	38	20
138	Haddock, breaded, fried	3 oz._____	85	66	140	17	5
139	Ocean perch, breaded, fried.	3 oz._____	85	59	195	16	11
140	Oysters, raw, meat only (13–19 med. selects).	1 cup_____	240	85	160	20	4
141	Salmon, pink, canned__	3 oz._____	85	71	120	17	5
142	Sardines, Atlantic, canned in oil, drained solids.	3 oz._____	85	62	175	20	9

EDIBLE PART OF FOODS (*continued*)

Fatty acids			Carbo-hydrate	Cal-cium	Iron	Vita-min A value	Thia-min	Ribo-flavin	Niacin	Ascor-bic acid
Satu-rated (total)	Unsaturated									
	Oleic	Lin-oleic								
Grams	Grams	Grams	Grams	Milli-grams	Milli-grams	Inter-national units	Milli-grams	Milli-grams	Milli-grams	Milli-grams
------	------	------	Trace	4	1.0	-------	.10	.07	1.5	------
------	------	------	Trace	3	.7	-------	.07	.07	1.2	------
------	------	------	Trace	1	.3	-------	.01	.02	.4	------
5	4	Trace	------	9	2.7	-------	.06	.21	4.6	------
7	6	Trace	0	10	2.9	-------	.11	.26	6.6	------
------	------	------	0	25	.6	40	.09	.08	1.6	------
------	------	------	2	59	5.2	90	.08	.15	1.1	8
------	------	------	2	47	3.5	-------	.01	.09	.9	------
------	------	------	1	38	.7	-------	.07	.07	1.6	------
5	4	10	15	25	0.9	-------	0.09	0.16	3.6	------
1	3	Trace	5	34	1.0	-------	.03	.06	2.7	2
------	------	------	6	28	1.1	-------	.08	.09	1.5	------
------	------	------	8	226	13.2	740	.33	.43	6.0	------
1	1	Trace	0	[4] 167	.7	60	.03	.16	6.8	------
------	------	------	0	372	2.5	190	.02	.17	4.6	------

TABLE 1.—NUTRITIVE VALUES OF THE

	Food, approximate measure, and weight (in grams)			Water	Food energy	Pro-tein	Fat
	MEAT, POULTRY, FISH, SHELLFISH; RELATED PRODUCTS—Continued						
	Fish and shellfish—Continued		*Grams*	*Per-cent*	*Calo-ries*	*Grams*	*Grams*
143	Shad, baked with table fat and bacon.	3 oz.	85	64	170	20	10
144	Shrimp, canned, meat	3 oz.	85	70	100	21	1
145	Swordfish, broiled with butter or margarine.	3 oz.	85	65	150	24	5
146	Tuna, canned in oil, drained solids.	3 oz.	85	61	170	24	7
	MATURE DRY BEANS AND PEAS, NUTS, PEANUTS; RELATED PRODUCTS						
147	Almonds, shelled, whole kernels.	1 cup	142	5	850	26	77
	Beans, dry:						
	Common varieties as Great Northern, navy, and others:						
	Cooked, drained:						
148	Great Northern	1 cup	180	69	210	14	1
149	Navy (pea)	1 cup	190	69	225	15	1
	Canned, solids and liquid:						
	White with—						
150	Frankfurters (sliced).	1 cup	255	71	365	19	18
151	Pork and tomato sauce.	1 cup	255	71	310	16	7
152	Pork and sweet sauce.	1 cup	255	66	385	16	12
153	Red kidney	1 cup	255	76	230	15	1
154	Lima, cooked, drained.	1 cup	190	64	260	16	1

[4]If bones are discarded, value will be greatly reduced.

Fatty acids			Carbo-hy-drate	Cal-cium	Iron	Vita-min A value	Thia-min	Ribo-flavin	Niacin	Ascor-bic acid
Satu-rated (total)	Unsaturated									
	Oleic	Lin-oleic								
Grams	*Grams*	*Grams*	*Grams*	*Milli-grams*	*Milli-grams*	*Inter-national units*	*Milli-grams*	*Milli-grams*	*Milli-grams*	*Milli-grams*
------	------	------	0	20	.5	20	.11	.22	7.3	------
------	------	------	1	98	2.6	50	.01	.03	1.5	------
------	------	------	0	23	1.1	1,750	.03	.04	9.3	------
2	1	1	0	7	1.6	70	.04	.10	10.1	------
6	52	15	28	332	6.7	0	.34	1.31	5.0	Trace
------	------	------	38	90	4.9	0	.25	.13	1.3	0
------	------	------	40	95	5.1	0	.27	.13	1.3	0
------	------	------	32	94	4.8	330	.18	.15	3.3	Trace
2	3	1	49	138	4.6	330	.20	.08	1.5	5
4	5	1	54	161	5.9	------	.15	.10	1.3	------
------	------	------	42	74	4.6	10	.13	.10	1.5	------
------	------	------	49	55	5.9	------	.25	.11	1.3	------

TABLE 1.—NUTRITIVE VALUES OF THE

	Food, approximate measure, and weight (in grams)			Water	Food energy	Pro-tein	Fat
	MATURE DRY BEANS AND PEAS, NUTS, PEANUTS; RELATED PRODUCTS—Con.						
			Grams	*Per-cent*	*Calo-ries*	*Grams*	*Gram*
155	Cashew nuts, roasted	1 cup	140	5	785	24	64
	Coconut, fresh, meat only:						
156	Pieces, approx. 2 by 2 by ½ inch.	1 piece	45	51	155	2	16
157	Shredded or grated, firmly packed.	1 cup	130	51	450	5	46
158	Cowpeas or blackeye peas, dry, cooked.	1 cup	248	80	190	13	1
159	Peanuts, roasted, salted, halves.	1 cup	144	2	840	37	72
160	Peanut butter	1 tbsp	16	2	95	4	8
161	Peas, split, dry, cooked	1 cup	250	70	290	20	1
162	Pecans, halves	1 cup	108	3	740	10	77
163	Walnuts, black or native, chopped.	1 cup	126	3	790	26	75
	VEGETABLES AND VEGETABLE PRODUCTS						
	Asparagus, green:						
	Cooked, drained:						
164	Spears, ½-in. diam. at base.	4 spears	60	94	10	1	Trace
165	Pieces, 1½ to 2-in. lengths.	1 cup	145	94	30	3	Trace
166	Canned, solids and liquid.	1 cup	244	94	45	5	1
	Beans:						
167	Lima, immature seeds, cooked, drained.	1 cup	170	71	190	13	1

Fatty acids			Carbohydrate	Calcium	Iron	Vitamin A value	Thiamin	Riboflavin	Niacin	Ascorbic acid
Saturated (total)	Unsaturated									
	Oleic	Linoleic								
Grams	*Grams*	*Grams*	*Grams*	*Milligrams*	*Milligrams*	*International units*	*Milligrams*	*Milligrams*	*Milligrams*	*Milligrams*
11	45	4	41	53	5.3	140	.60	.35	2.5	------
14	1	Trace	4	6	.8	0	.02	.01	.2	1
39	3	Trace	12	17	2.2	0	.07	.03	.7	4
------	------	------	34	42	3.2	20	.41	.11	1.1	Trace
16	31	21	27	107	3.0	------	.46	.19	24.7	0
2	4	2	3	9	.3	------	.02	.02	2.4	0
			52	28	4.2	100	.37	.22	2.2	------
5	48	15	16	79	2.6	140	.93	.14	1.0	2
4	26	36	19	Trace	7.6	380	.28	.14	.9	------
------	------	------	2	13	.4	540	.10	.11	.8	16
------	------	------	5	30	.9	1,310	.23	.26	2.0	38
------	------	------	7	44	4.1	1,240	.15	.22	2.0	37
------	------	------	34	80	4.3	480	.31	.17	2.2	29

TABLE 1.—NUTRITIVE VALUES OF THE

	Food, approximate measure, and weight (in grams)			Water	Food energy	Protein	Fat
	VEGETABLES AND VEGETABLE PRODUCTS—Continued						
	Beans—Continued		*Grams*	*Percent*	*Calories*	*Grams*	*Grams*
	Snap:						
	Green:						
168	Cooked, drained___	1 cup_____	125	92	30	2	Trace
169	Canned, solids and liquid.	1 cup_____	239	94	45	2	Trace
	Yellow or wax:						
170	Cooked, drained___	1 cup_____	125	93	30	2	Trace
171	Canned, solids and liquid.	1 cup_____	239	94	45	2	1
172	Sprouted mung beans, cooked, drained.	1 cup_____	125	91	35	4	Trace
	Beets:						
	Cooked, drained, peeled:						
173	Whole beets, 2-in. diam.	2 beets_____	100	91	30	1	Trace
174	Diced or sliced_____	1 cup_____	170	91	55	2	Trace
175	Canned, solids and liquid.	1 cup_____	246	90	85	2	Trace
176	Beet greens, leaves and stems, cooked, drained.	1 cup_____	145	94	25	3	Trace
	Blackeye peas. See Cowpeas.						
	Broccoli, cooked, drained:						
177	Whole stalks, medium size.	1 stalk_____	180	91	45	6	1
178	Stalks cut into ½-in. pieces.	1 cup_____	155	91	40	5	1
179	Chopped, yield from 10-oz. frozen pkg.	1⅜ cups____	250	92	65	7	1

EDIBLE PART OF FOODS *(continued)*

Fatty acids			Carbo-hydrate	Cal-cium	Iron	Vita-min A value	Thia-min	Ribo-flavin	Niacin	Ascor-bic acid
Satu-rated (total)	Unsaturated									
	Oleic	Lin-oleic								
Grams	Grams	Grams	Grams	Milli-grams	Milli-grams	Inter-national units	Milli-grams	Milli-grams	Milli-grams	Milli-grams
------	------	------	7	63	.8	680	.09	.11	.6	15
------	------	------	10	81	2.9	690	.07	.10	.7	10
------	------	------	6	63	0.8	290	0.09	0.11	0.6	16
------	------	------	10	81	2.9	140	.07	.10	.7	12
------	------	------	7	21	1.1	30	.11	.13	.9	8
------	------	------	7	14	.5	20	.03	.04	.3	6
------	------	------	12	24	.9	30	.05	.07	.5	10
------	------	------	19	34	1.5	20	.02	.05	.2	7
------	------	------	5	144	2.8	7,400	.10	.22	.4	22
------	------	------	8	158	1.4	4,500	.16	.36	1.4	162
------	------	------	7	136	1.2	3,880	.14	.31	1.2	140
------	------	------	12	135	1.8	6,500	.15	.30	1.3	143

TABLE 1.—NUTRITIVE VALUES OF THE

Food, approximate measure, and weight (in grams)			Water	Food energy	Pro- tein	Fat

VEGETABLES AND VEGETABLE PRODUCTS—Continued

				Per- cent	Calo- ries	Grams	Grams
			Grams				
180	Brussels sprouts, 7–8 sprouts (1¼ to 1½ in. diam.) per cup, cooked.	1 cup_____	155	88	55	7	1
	Cabbage:						
	Common varieties:						
	Raw:						
181	Coarsely shredded or sliced.	1 cup_____	70	92	15	1	Trace
182	Finely shredded or chopped.	1 cup_____	90	92	20	1	Trace
183	Cooked_____	1 cup_____	145	94	30	2	Trace
184	Red, raw, coarsely shredded.	1 cup_____	70	90	20	1	Trace
185	Savoy, raw, coarsely shredded.	1 cup_____	70	92	15	2	Trace
186	Cabbage, celery or Chinese, raw, cut in 1-in. pieces.	1 cup_____	75	95	10	1	Trace
187	Cabbage, spoon (or pakchoy), cooked.	1 cup_____	170	95	25	2	Trace
	Carrots:						
	Raw:						
188	Whole, 5½ by 1 inch, (25 thin strips).	1 carrot_____	50	88	20	1	Trace
189	Grated_____	1 cup_____	110	88	45	1	Trace
190	Cooked, diced_____	1 cup_____	145	91	45	1	Trace
191	Canned, strained or chopped (baby food).	1 ounce_____	28	92	10	Trace	Trace
192	Cauliflower, cooked, flowerbuds.	1 cup_____	120	93	25	3	Trace

EDIBLE PART OF FOODS *(continued)*

Fatty acids			Carbo-hy-drate	Cal-cium	Iron	Vita-min A value	Thia-min	Ribo-flavin	Niacin	Ascor-bic acid
Satu-rated (total)	Unsaturated									
	Oleic	Lin-oleic								
Grams	*Grams*	*Grams*	*Grams*	*Milli-grams*	*Milli-grams*	*Inter-national units*	*Milli-grams*	*Milli-grams*	*Milli-grams*	*Milli-grams*
------	------	------	10	50	1.7	810	.12	.22	1.2	135
------	------	------	4	34	.3	90	.04	.04	.2	33
------	------	------	5	44	.4	120	.05	.05	.3	42
------	------	------	6	64	.4	190	.06	.06	.4	48
------	------	------	5	29	.6	30	.06	.04	.3	43
------	------	------	3	47	.6	140	.04	.06	.2	39
------	------	------	2	32	.5	110	.04	.03	.5	19
------	------	------	4	252	1.0	5,270	.07	.14	1.2	26
------	------	------	5	18	.4	5,500	.03	.03	.3	4
------	------	------	11	41	.8	12,100	.06	.06	.7	9
------	------	------	10	48	.9	15,220	.08	.07	.7	9
------	------	------	2	7	.1	3,690	.01	.01	.1	1
------	------	------	5	25	.8	70	.11	.10	.7	66

TABLE 1.—NUTRITIVE VALUES OF THE

	Food, approximate measure, and weight (in grams)			Water	Food energy	Pro-tein	Fat
	VEGETABLES AND VEGETABLE PRODUCTS—Continued						
			Grams	*Per-cent*	*Calo-ries*	*Grams*	*Grams*
	Celery, raw:						
193	Stalk, large outer, 8 by about 1½ inches, at root end.	1 stalk	40	94	5	Trace	Trace
194	Pieces, diced	1 cup	100	94	15	1	Trace
195	Collards, cooked	1 cup	190	91	55	5	1
	Corn, sweet:						
196	Cooked, ear 5 by 1¾ inches.[5]	1 ear	140	74	70	3	1
197	Canned, solids and liquid.	1 cup	256	81	170	5	2
198	Cowpeas, cooked, immature seeds.	1 cup	160	72	175	13	1
	Cucumbers, 10-ounce; 7½ by about 2 inches:						
199	Raw, pared	1 cucumber	207	96	30	1	Trace
200	Raw, pared, center slice ⅛-inch thick.	6 slices	50	96	5	Trace	Trace
201	Dandelion greens, cooked	1 cup	180	90	60	4	1
202	Endive, curly (including escarole).	2 ounces	57	93	10	1	Trace
203	Kale, leaves including stems, cooked.	1 cup	110	91	30	4	1
	Lettuce, raw:						
204	Butterhead, as Boston types; head, 4-inch diameter.	1 head	220	95	30	3	Trace
205	Crisphead, as Iceberg; head, 4¾-inch diameter.	1 head	454	96	60	4	Trace
206	Looseleaf, or bunching varieties, leaves.	2 large	50	94	10	1	Trace

[5]Measure and weight apply to entire vegetable or fruit including parts not usually eaten.

EDIBLE PART OF FOODS *(continued)*

Fatty acids			Carbohydrate	Calcium	Iron	Vitamin A value	Thiamin	Riboflavin	Niacin	Ascorbic acid
Saturated (total)	Unsaturated									
	Oleic	Linoleic								
Grams	*Grams*	*Grams*	*Grams*	*Milligrams*	*Milligrams*	*International units*	*Milligrams*	*Milligrams*	*Milligrams*	*Milligrams*
------	------	------	2	16	.1	100	.01	.01	.1	4
------	------	------	4	39	.3	240	.03	.03	.3	9
------	------	------	9	289	1.1	10,260	.27	.37	2.4	87
------	------	------	16	2	.5	[6]310	.09	.08	1.0	7
------	------	------	40	10	1.0	[6]690	.07	.12	2.3	13
------	------	------	29	38	3.4	560	.49	.18	2.3	28
------	------	------	7	35	.6	Trace	.07	.09	.4	23
------	------	------	2	8	.2	Trace	.02	.02	.1	6
------	------	------	12	252	3.2	21,060	.24	.29	------	32
------	------	------	2	46	1.0	1,870	0.04	0.08	0.3	6
------	------	------	4	147	1.3	8,140	------	------	------	68
------	------	------	6	77	4.4	2,130	.14	.13	.6	18
------	------	------	13	91	2.3	1,500	.29	.27	1.3	29
------	------	------	2	34	.7	950	.03	.04	.2	9

[6]Based on yellow varieties; white varieties contain only a trace of cryptoxanthin and carotenes, the pigments in corn that have biological activity.

TABLE 1.—NUTRITIVE VALUES OF THE

	Food, approximate measure, and weight (in grams)			Water	Food energy	Pro-tein	Fat
	VEGETABLES AND VEGETABLE PRODUCTS—Continued						
			Grams	Per-cent	Calo-ries	Grams	Grams
207	Mushrooms, canned, solids and liquid.	1 cup	244	93	40	5	Trace
208	Mustard greens, cooked	1 cup	140	93	35	3	1
209	Okra, cooked, pod 3 by ⅝ inch.	8 pods	85	91	25	2	Trace
	Onions:						
	Mature:						
210	Raw, onion 2½-inch diameter.	1 onion	110	89	40	2	Trace
211	Cooked	1 cup	210	92	60	3	Trace
212	Young green, small, without tops.	6 onions	50	88	20	1	Trace
213	Parsley, raw, chopped	1 tablespoon	4	85	Trace	Trace	Trace
214	Parsnips, cooked	1 cup	155	82	100	2	1
	Peas, green:						
215	Cooked	1 cup	160	82	115	9	1
216	Canned, solids and liquid.	1 cup	249	83	165	9	1
217	Canned, strained (baby food).	1 ounce	28	86	15	1	Trace
218	Peppers, hot, red, without seeds, dried (ground chili powder, added seasonings).	1 tablespoon	15	8	50	2	2
	Peppers, sweet:						
	Raw, about 5 per pound:						
219	Green pod without stem and seeds.	1 pod	74	93	15	1	Trace
220	Cooked, boiled, drained	1 pod	73	95	15	1	Trace

Fatty acids			Carbo-hy-drate	Cal-cium	Iron	Vita-min A value	Thia-min	Ribo-flavin	Niacin	Ascor-bic acid
Satu-rated (total)	Unsaturated									
	Oleic	Lin-oleic								
Grams	Grams	Grams	Grams	Milli-grams	Milli-grams	Inter-national units	Milli-grams	Milli-grams	Milli-grams	Milli-grams
-----	-----	-----	6	15	1.2	Trace	.04	.60	4.8	4
-----	-----	-----	6	193	2.5	8,120	.11	.19	.9	68
-----	-----	-----	5	78	.4	420	.11	.15	.8	17
-----	-----	-----	10	30	.6	40	.04	.04	.2	11
-----	-----	-----	14	50	.8	80	.06	.06	.4	14
-----	-----	-----	5	20	.3	Trace	.02	.02	.2	12
-----	-----	-----	Trace	8	.2	340	Trace	.01	Trace	7
-----	-----	-----	23	70	.9	50	.11	.12	.2	16
-----	-----	-----	19	37	2.9	860	.44	.17	3.7	33
-----	-----	-----	31	50	4.2	1,120	.23	.13	2.2	22
-----	-----	-----	3	3	.4	140	.02	.02	.4	3
-----	-----	-----	8	40	2.3	9,750	.03	.17	1.3	2
-----	-----	-----	4	7	.5	310	.06	.06	.4	94
-----	-----	-----	3	7	.4	310	.05	.05	.4	70

TABLE 1.—NUTRITIVE VALUES OF THE

	Food, approximate measure, and weight (in grams)			Water	Food energy	Protein	Fat
	VEGETABLES AND VEGETABLE PRODUCTS—Continued						
			Grams	Percent	Calories	Grams	Grams
	Potatoes, medium (about 3 per pound raw):						
221	Baked, peeled after baking.	1 potato_____	99	75	90	3	Trace
	Boiled:						
222	Peeled after boiling__	1 potato_____	136	80	105	3	Trace
223	Peeled before boiling_	1 potato_____	122	83	80	2	Trace
	French-fried, piece 2 by ½ by ½ inch:						
224	Cooked in deep fat____	10 pieces____	57	45	155	2	7
225	Frozen, heated_____	10 pieces____	57	53	125	2	5
	Mashed:						
226	Milk added_____	1 cup_____	195	83	125	4	1
227	Milk and butter added.	1 cup_____	195	80	185	4	8
228	Potato chips, medium, 2-inch diameter.	10 chips_____	20	2	115	1	8
229	Pumpkin, canned_____	1 cup_____	228	90	75	2	1
230	Radishes, raw, small, without tops.	4 radishes___	40	94	5	Trace	Trace
231	Sauerkraut, canned, solids and liquid.	1 cup_____	235	93	45	2	Trace
	Spinach:						
232	Cooked_____	1 cup_____	180	92	40	5	1
233	Canned, drained solids_	1 cup_____	180	91	45	5	1
	Squash:						
	Cooked:						
234	Summer, diced_____	1 cup_____	210	96	30	2	Trace
235	Winter, baked, mashed.	1 cup_____	205	81	130	4	1
	Sweetpotatoes:						
	Cooked, medium, 5 by 2 inches, weight raw about 6 ounces:						

Fatty acids			Carbohydrate	Calcium	Iron	Vitamin A value	Thiamin	Riboflavin	Niacin	Ascorbic acid
Saturated (total)	Unsaturated									
	Oleic	Linoleic								
Grams	Grams	Grams	Grams	Milligrams	Milligrams	International units	Milligrams	Milligrams	Milligrams	Milligrams
------	------	------	21	9	.7	Trace	.10	.04	1.7	20
------	------	------	23	10	.8	Trace	.13	.05	2.0	22
------	------	------	18	7	.6	Trace	.11	.04	1.4	20
2	2	4	20	9	.7	Trace	.07	.04	1.8	12
1	1	2	19	5	1.0	Trace	.08	.01	1.5	12
------	------	------	25	47	.8	50	.16	.10	2.0	19
4	3	Trace	24	47	.8	330	.16	.10	1.9	18
2	2	4	10	8	.4	Trace	.04	.01	1.0	3
------	------	------	18	57	.9	14,590	.07	.12	1.3	12
------	------	------	1	12	.4	Trace	.01	.01	.1	10
------	------	------	9	85	1.2	120	.07	.09	.4	33
------	------	------	6	167	4.0	14,580	.13	.25	1.0	50
------	------	------	6	212	4.7	14,400	.03	.21	.6	24
------	------	------	7	52	.8	820	.10	.16	1.6	21
------	------	------	32	57	1.6	8,610	.10	.27	1.4	27

TABLE 1.—NUTRITIVE VALUES OF THE

	Food, approximate measure, and weight (in grams)		Water	Food energy	Pro-tein	Fat
		Grams	Per-cent	Calo-ries	Grams	Grams

VEGETABLES AND VEGETABLE PRODUCTS—Continued

	Food, approximate measure, and weight (in grams)		Water	Food energy	Pro-tein	Fat
	Sweetpotatoes—Continued					
236	Baked, peeled after baking.	1 sweet-potato. 110	64	155	2	1
237	Boiled, peeled after boiling.	1 sweet-potato. 147	71	170	2	1
238	Candied, 3½ by 2¼ inches.	1 sweet-potato. 175	60	295	2	6
239	Canned, vacuum or solid pack.	1 cup_____ 218	72	235	4	Trace
	Tomatoes:					
240	Raw, approx. 3-in. diam. 2⅛ in. high; wt., 7 oz.	1 tomato____ 200	94	40	2	Trace
241	Canned, solids and liquid.	1 cup_____ 241	94	50	2	1
	Tomato catsup:					
242	Cup_____	1 cup_____ 273	69	290	6	1
243	Tablespoon_____	1 tbsp._____ 15	69	15	Trace	Trace
	Tomato juice, canned:					
244	Cup_____	1 cup_____ 243	94	45	2	Trace
245	Glass (6 fl. oz.)_____	1 glass_____ 182	94	35	2	Trace
246	Turnips, cooked, diced___	1 cup_____ 155	94	35	1	Trace
247	Turnip greens, cooked____	1 cup_____ 145	94	30	3	Trace

FRUITS AND FRUIT PRODUCTS

248	Apples, raw (about 3 per lb.).[5]	1 apple_____ 150	85	70	Trace	Trace
249	Apple juice, bottled or canned.	1 cup_____ 248	88	120	Trace	Trace
	Applesauce, canned:					
250	Sweetened_____	1 cup_____ 255	76	230	1	Trace

[5]Measure and weight apply to entire vegetable or fruit including parts not usually eaten.

EDIBLE PART OF FOODS *(continued)*

Fatty acids			Carbo-hy-drate	Cal-cium	Iron	Vita-min A value	Thia-min	Ribo-flavin	Niacin	Ascor-bic acid
Satu-rated (total)	Unsaturated									
	Oleic	Lin-oleic								
Grams	*Grams*	*Grams*	*Grams*	*Milli-grams*	*Milli-grams*	*Inter-national units*	*Milli-grams*	*Milli-grams*	*Milli-grams*	*Milli-grams*
------	------	------	36	44	1.0	8,910	.10	.07	.7	24
------	------	------	39	47	1.0	11,610	.13	.09	.9	25
2	3	1	60	65	1.6	11,030	0.10	0.08	0.8	17
------	------	------	54	54	1.7	17,000	.10	.10	1.4	30
------	------	------	9	24	.9	1,640	.11	.07	1.3	[7] 42
------	------	------	10	14	1.2	2,170	.12	.07	1.7	41
------	------	------	69	60	2.2	3,820	.25	.19	4.4	41
------	------	------	4	3	.1	210	.01	.01	.2	2
------	------	------	10	17	2.2	1,940	.12	.07	1.9	39
------	------	------	8	13	1.6	1,460	.09	.05	1.5	29
------	------	------	8	54	.6	Trace	.06	.08	.5	34
------	------	------	5	252	1.5	8,270	.15	.33	.7	68
------	------	------	18	8	.4	50	.04	.02	.1	3
------	------	------	30	15	1.5	------	.02	.05	.2	2
------	------	------	61	10	1.3	100	.05	.03	.1	[8] 3

[7]Year-round average. Samples marketed from November through May, average 20 milligrams per 200-gram tomato; from June through October, around 52 milligrams.

TABLE 1.—NUTRITIVE VALUES OF THE

	Food, approximate measure, and weight (in grams)			Water	Food energy	Protein	Fat
	FRUITS AND FRUIT PRODUCTS—Con.						
	Applesauce, canned —Continued		*Grams*	*Per-cent*	*Calo-ries*	*Grams*	*Grams*
251	Unsweetened or artificially sweetened.	1 cup_____	244	88	100	1	Trace
	Apricots:						
252	Raw (about 12 per lb.) [5]	3 apricots____	114	85	55	1	Trace
253	Canned in heavy sirup__	1 cup_____	259	77	220	2	Trace
254	Dried, uncooked (40 halves per cup).	1 cup_____	150	25	390	8	1
255	Cooked, unsweetened, fruit and liquid.	1 cup_____	285	76	240	5	1
256	Apricot nectar, canned___	1 cup_____	251	85	140	1	Trace
	Avocados, whole fruit, raw: [5]						
257	California (mid- and late-winter; diam. 3⅛ in.).	1 avocado___	284	74	370	5	37
258	Florida (late summer, fall; diam. 3⅝ in.).	1 avocado___	454	78	390	4	33
259	Bananas, raw, medium size.[5]	1 banana____	175	76	100	1	Trace
260	Banana flakes_____	1 cup_____	100	3	340	4	1
261	Blackberries, raw_____	1 cup_____	144	84	85	2	1
262	Blueberries, raw_____	1 cup_____	140	83	85	1	1
263	Cantaloups, raw; medium, 5-inch diameter about 1⅔ pounds.[5]	½ melon____	385	91	60	1	Trace
264	Cherries, canned, red, sour, pitted, water pack.	1 cup_____	244	88	105	2	Trace
265	Cranberry juice cocktail, canned.	1 cup_____	250	83	165	Trace	Trace

[5]Measure and weight apply to entire vegetable or fruit including parts not usually eaten.

[8]This is the amount from the fruit. Additional ascorbic acid may be added by the manufacturer. Refer to the label for this information.

EDIBLE PART OF FOODS *(continued)*

Fatty acids			Carbohydrate	Calcium	Iron	Vitamin A value	Thiamin	Riboflavin	Niacin	Ascorbic acid
Saturated (total)	Unsaturated									
	Oleic	Linoleic								
Grams	*Grams*	*Grams*	*Grams*	*Milligrams*	*Milligrams*	*International units*	*Milligrams*	*Milligrams*	*Milligrams*	*Milligrams*
-----	-----	-----	26	10	1.2	100	.05	.02	.1	[8] 2
-----	-----	-----	14	18	.5	2,890	.03	.04	.7	10
-----	-----	-----	57	28	.8	4,510	.05	.06	.9	10
-----	-----	-----	100	100	8.2	16,350	.02	.23	4.9	19
-----	-----	-----	62	63	5.1	8,550	.01	.13	2.8	8
-----	-----	-----	37	23	.5	2,380	.03	.03	.5	[8] 8
7	17	5	13	22	1.3	630	.24	.43	3.5	30
7	15	4	27	30	1.8	880	.33	.61	4.9	43
-----	-----	-----	26	10	.8	230	.06	.07	.8	12
-----	-----	-----	89	32	2.8	760	.18	.24	2.8	7
-----	-----	-----	19	46	1.3	290	.05	.06	.5	30
-----	-----	-----	21	21	1.4	140	.04	.08	.6	20
-----	-----	-----	14	27	.8	[9] 6,540	.08	.06	1.2	63
-----	-----	-----	26	37	.7	1,660	.07	.05	.5	12
-----	-----	-----	42	13	.8	Trace	.03	.03	.1	[10] 40

[9]Value for varieties with orange-colored flesh; value for varieties with green flesh would be about 540 I.U.

[10]Value listed is based on products with label stating 30 milligrams per 6 fl. oz. serving.

TABLE 1.—NUTRITIVE VALUES OF THE

	Food, approximate measure, and weight (in grams)			Water	Food energy	Pro-tein	Fat
	FRUITS AND FRUIT PRODUCTS—Con.						
			Grams	*Per-cent*	*Calo-ries*	*Grams*	*Grams*
266	Cranberry sauce, sweet-ened, canned, strained.	1 cup	277	62	405	Trace	1
267	Dates, pitted, cut	1 cup	178	22	490	4	1
268	Figs, dried, large, 2 by 1 in.	1 fig	21	23	60	1	Trace
269	Fruit cocktail, canned, in heavy sirup.	1 cup	256	80	195	1	Trace
	Grapefruit:						
	Raw, medium, 3¾-in. diam.[5]						
270	White	½ grape-fruit.	241	89	45	1	Trace
271	Pink or red	½ grape-fruit.	241	89	50	1	Trace
272	Canned, sirup pack	1 cup	254	81	180	2	Trace
	Grapefruit juice:						
273	Fresh	1 cup	246	90	95	1	Trace
	Canned, white:						
274	Unsweetened	1 cup	247	89	100	1	Trace
275	Sweetened	1 cup	250	86	130	1	Trace
	Frozen, concentrate, unsweetened:						
276	Undiluted, can, 6 fluid ounces.	1 can	207	62	300	4	1
277	Diluted with 3 parts water, by volume.	1 cup	247	89	100	1	Trace
278	Dehydrated crystals	4 oz.	113	1	410	6	1
279	Prepared with water (1 pound yields about 1 gallon).	1 cup	247	90	100	1	Trace

[5]Measure and weight apply to entire vegetable or fruit including parts not usually eaten.

EDIBLE PART OF FOODS *(continued)*

Fatty acids			Carbo-hy-drate	Cal-cium	Iron	Vita-min A value	Thia-min	Ribo-flavin	Niacin	Ascor-bic acid
Satu-rated (total)	Unsaturated									
	Oleic	Lin-oleic								
Grams	Grams	Grams	Grams	Milli-grams	Milli-grams	Inter-national units	Milli-grams	Milli-grams	Milli-grams	Milli-grams
------	------	------	104	17	.6	60	.03	.03	.1	6
------	------	------	130	105	5.3	90	.16	.17	3.9	0
------	------	------	15	26	.6	20	.02	.02	.1	0
------	------	------	50	23	1.0	360	.05	.03	1.3	5
------	------	------	12	19	0.5	10	0.05	0.02	0.2	44
------	------	------	13	20	0.5	540	0.05	0.02	0.2	44
------	------	------	45	33	.8	30	.08	.05	.5	76
------	------	------	23	22	.5	(11)	.09	.04	.4	92
------	------	------	24	20	1.0	20	.07	.04	.4	84
------	------	------	32	20	1.0	20	.07	.04	.4	78
------	------	------	72	70	.8	60	.29	.12	1.4	286
------	------	------	24	25	.2	20	.10	.04	.5	96
------	------	------	102	100	1.2	80	.40	.20	2.0	396
------	------	------	24	22	.2	20	.10	.05	.5	91

[11]For white-fleshed varieties value is about 20 I.U. per cup; for red-fleshed varieties, 1,080 I.U. per cup.

TABLE 1.—NUTRITIVE VALUES OF THE

Food, approximate measure, and weight (in grams)			Water	Food energy	Pro-tein	Fat

FRUITS AND FRUIT PRODUCTS—Con.

				Grams	Per-cent	Calo-ries	Grams	Grams
	Grapes, raw: [5]							
280	American type (slip skin).	1 cup		153	82	65	1	1
281	European type (adherent skin).	1 cup		160	81	95	1	Trace
	Grapejuice:							
282	Canned or bottled	1 cup		253	83	165	1	Trace
	Frozen concentrate, sweetened:							
283	Undiluted, can, 6 fluid ounces.	1 can		216	53	395	1	Trace
284	Diluted with 3 parts water, by volume.	1 cup		250	86	135	1	Trace
285	Grapejuice drink, canned	1 cup		250	86	135	Trace	Trace
286	Lemons, raw, 2⅛-in. diam., size 165.[5] Used for juice.	1 lemon		110	90	20	1	Trace
287	Lemon juice, raw	1 cup		244	91	60	1	Trace
	Lemonade concentrate:							
288	Frozen, 6 fl. oz. per can	1 can		219	48	430	Trace	Trace
289	Diluted with 4⅓ parts water, by volume.	1 cup		248	88	110	Trace	Trace
	Lime juice:							
290	Fresh	1 cup		246	90	65	1	Trace
291	Canned, unsweetened	1 cup		246	90	65	1	Trace
	Limeade concentrate, frozen:							
292	Undiluted, can, 6 fluid ounces.	1 can		218	50	410	Trace	Trace
293	Diluted with 4⅓ parts water, by volume.	1 cup		247	90	100	Trace	Trace

[5]Measure and weight apply to entire vegetable or fruit including parts not usually eaten.

EDIBLE PART OF FOODS *(continued)*

Fatty acids			Carbo-hy-drate	Cal-cium	Iron	Vita-min A value	Thia-min	Ribo-flavin	Niacin	Ascor-bic acid
Satu-rated (total)	Unsaturated									
	Oleic	Lin-oleic								
Grams	Grams	Grams	Grams	Milli-grams	Milli-grams	Inter-national units	Milli-grams	Milli-grams	Milli-grams	Milli-grams
------	------	------	15	15	.4	100	.05	.03	.2	3
------	------	------	25	17	.6	140	.07	.04	.4	6
------	------	------	42	28	.8	-------	.10	.05	.5	Trace
------	------	------	100	22	.9	40	.13	.22	1.5	(12)
------	------	------	33	8	.3	10	.05	.08	.5	(12)
------	------	------	35	8	.3	-------	.03	.03	.3	(12)
------	------	------	6	19	.4	10	.03	.01	.1	39
------	------	------	20	17	.5	50	.07	.02	.2	112
------	------	------	112	9	.4	40	.04	.07	.7	66
------	------	------	28	2	Trace	Trace	Trace	.02	.2	17
------	------	------	22	22	.5	20	.05	.02	.2	79
------	------	------	22	22	.5	20	.05	.02	.2	52
------	------	------	108	11	.2	Trace	.02	.02	.2	26
------	------	------	27	2	Trace	Trace	Trace	Trace	Trace	5

[12]Present only if added by the manufacturer. Refer to the label for this information.

TABLE 1.—NUTRITIVE VALUES OF THE

	Food, approximate measure, and weight (in grams)			Water	Food energy	Protein	Fat
	FRUITS AND FRUIT PRODUCTS—Con.						
			Grams	*Percent*	*Calories*	*Grams*	*Grams*
294	Oranges, raw, 2⅝-in. diam., all commercial, varieties.[5]	1 orange	180	86	65	1	Trace
295	Orange juice, fresh, all varieties.	1 cup	248	88	110	2	1
296	Canned, unsweetened	1 cup	249	87	120	2	Trace
	Frozen concentrate:						
297	Undiluted, can, 6 fluid ounces.	1 can	213	55	360	5	Trace
298	Diluted with 3 parts water, by volume.	1 cup	249	87	120	2	Trace
299	Dehydrated crystals	4 oz.	113	1	430	6	2
300	Prepared with water (1 pound yields about 1 gallon).	1 cup	248	88	115	2	1
301	Orange-apricot juice drink	1 cup	249	87	125	1	Trace
	Orange and grapefruit juice:						
	Frozen concentrate:						
302	Undiluted, can, 6 fluid ounces.	1 can	210	59	330	4	1
303	Diluted with 3 parts water, by volume.	1 cup	248	88	110	1	Trace
304	Papayas, raw, ½-inch cubes.	1 cup	182	89	70	1	Trace
	Peaches:						
	Raw:						
305	Whole, medium, 2-inch diameter, about 4 per pound.[5]	1 peach	114	89	35	1	Trace

[5]Measure and weight apply to entire vegetable or fruit including parts not usually eaten.

[10]Value listed is based on product with label stating 30 milligrams per 6 fl. oz. serving.

EDIBLE PART OF FOODS *(continued)*

Fatty acids			Carbohydrate	Calcium	Iron	Vitamin A value	Thiamin	Riboflavin	Niacin	Ascorbic acid
Saturated (total)	Unsaturated									
	Oleic	Linoleic								
Grams	Grams	Grams	Grams	Milligrams	Milligrams	International units	Milligrams	Milligrams	Milligrams	Milligrams
------	------	------	16	54	.5	260	.13	.05	.5	66
------	------	------	26	27	.5	500	.22	.07	1.0	124
------	------	------	28	25	1.0	500	.17	.05	.7	100
------	------	------	87	75	.9	1,620	.68	.11	2.8	360
------	------	------	29	25	.2	550	.22	.02	1.0	120
------	------	------	100	95	1.9	1,900	.76	.24	3.3	408
------	------	------	27	25	.5	500	.20	.07	1.0	109
------	------	------	32	12	.2	1,440	.05	.02	.5	[10] 40
------	------	------	78	61	0.8	800	0.48	0.06	2.3	302
------	------	------	26	20	.2	270	.16	.02	.8	102
------	------	------	18	36	.5	3,190	.07	.08	.5	102
------	------	------	10	9	.5	[13]1,320	.02	.05	1.0	7

[13]Based on yellow-fleshed varieties; for white-fleshed varieties value is about 50 I.U. per 114-gram peach and 80 I.U. per cup of sliced peaches.

TABLE 1.—NUTRITIVE VALUES OF THE

	Food, approximate measure, and weight (in grams)			Water	Food energy	Pro-tein	Fat
	FRUITS AND FRUIT PRODUCTS—Con.						
	Peaches—Continued			*Per-cent*	*Calo-ries*	*Grams*	*Grams*
	Raw—Continued		*Grams*				
306	Sliced_____	1 cup_____	168	89	65	1	Trace
	Canned, yellow-fleshed, solids and liquid:						
	Sirup pack, heavy:						
307	Halves or slices____	1 cup_____	257	79	200	1	Trace
308	Water pack_____	1 cup_____	245	91	75	1	Trace
309	Dried, uncooked_____	1 cup_____	160	25	420	5	1
310	Cooked, unsweet-ened, 10–12 halves and juice.	1 cup_____	270	77	220	3	1
	Frozen:						
311	Carton, 12 ounces, not thawed.	1 carton_____	340	76	300	1	Trace
	Pears:						
312	Raw, 3 by 2½-inch diameter.[5]	1 pear_____	182	83	100	1	1
	Canned, solids and liquid:						
	Sirup pack, heavy:						
313	Halves or slices____	1 cup_____	255	80	195	1	1
	Pineapple:						
314	Raw, diced_____	1 cup_____	140	85	75	1	Trace
	Canned, heavy sirup pack, solids and liquid:						
315	Crushed_____	1 cup_____	260	80	195	1	Trace
316	Sliced, slices and juice.	2 small or 1 large.	122	80	90	Trace	Trace
317	Pineapple juice, canned___	1 cup_____	249	86	135	1	Trace
	Plums, all except prunes:						
318	Raw, 2-inch diameter, about 2 ounces.[5]	1 plum_____	60	87	25	Trace	Trace
	Canned, sirup pack (Italian prunes):						
319	Plums (with pits) and juice.[5]	1 cup_____	256	77	205	1	Trace

[5]Measure and weight apply to entire vegetable or fruit including parts not usually eaten.

[8]This is the amount from the fruit. Additional ascorbic acid may be added by the manufacturer. Refer to the label for this information.

EDIBLE PART OF FOODS (continued)

Fatty acids			Carbo-hy-drate	Cal-cium	Iron	Vita-min A value	Thia-min	Ribo-flavin	Niacin	Ascor-bic acid
Satu-rated (total)	Unsaturated									
	Oleic	Lin-oleic								
Grams	Grams	Grams	Grams	Milli-grams	Milli-grams	Inter-national units	Milli-grams	Milli-grams	Milli-grams	Milli-grams
------	------	------	16	15	.8	[13]2,230	.03	.08	1.6	12
------	------	------	52	10	.8	1,100	.02	.06	1.4	7
------	------	------	20	10	.7	1,100	.02	.06	1.4	7
------	------	------	109	77	9.6	6,240	.02	.31	8.5	28
------	------	------	58	41	5.1	3,290	.01	.15	4.2	6
------	------	------	77	14	1.7	2,210	.03	.14	2.4	[14]135
------	------	------	25	13	.5	30	.04	.07	.2	7
------	------	------	50	13	.5	Trace	.03	.05	.3	4
------	------	------	19	24	.7	100	.12	.04	.3	24
------	------	------	50	29	.8	120	.20	.06	.5	17
------	------	------	24	13	.4	50	.09	.03	.2	8
------	------	------	34	37	.7	120	.12	.04	.5	[8]22
------	------	------	7	7	.3	140	.02	.02	.3	3
------	------	------	53	22	2.2	2,970	.05	.05	.9	4

[13]Based on yellow-fleshed varieties; for white-fleshed varieties value is about 50 I.U. per 114-gram peach and 80 I.U. per cup of sliced peaches.

[14]This value includes ascorbic acid added by manufacturer.

TABLE 1.—NUTRITIVE VALUES OF THE

	Food, approximate measure, and weight (in grams)		Water	Food energy	Pro-tein	Fat
		Grams	*Per-cent*	*Calo-ries*	*Grams*	*Grams*
	FRUITS AND FRUIT PRODUCTS—Con.					
	Prunes, dried, "softenized", medium:					
320	Uncooked [5]_____ 4 prunes_____	32	28	70	1	Trace
321	Cooked, unsweetened, 1 cup_____ 17–18 prunes and ⅓ cup liquid.[5]	270	66	295	2	1
322	Prune juice, canned or 1 cup_____ bottled.	256	80	200	1	Trace
	Raisins, seedless:					
323	Packaged, ½ oz. or 1 pkg._____ 1½ tbsp. per pkg.	14	18	40	Trace	Trace
324	Cup, pressed down_____ 1 cup_____	165	18	480	4	Trace
	Raspberries, red:					
325	Raw_____ 1 cup_____	123	84	70	1	1
326	Frozen, 10-ounce car- 1 carton_____ ton, not thawed.	284	74	275	2	1
327	Rhubarb, cooked, sugar 1 cup_____ added.	272	63	385	1	Trace
	Strawberries:					
328	Raw, capped_____ 1 cup_____	149	90	55	1	1
329	Frozen, 10-ounce car- 1 carton_____ ton, not thawed.	284	71	310	1	1
330	Tangerines, raw, medium, 1 tangerine__ 2⅜-in. diam., size 176.[5]	116	87	40	1	Trace
331	Tangerine juice, canned, 1 cup_____ sweetened.	249	87	125	1	1
332	Watermelon, raw, wedge, 1 wedge_____ 4 by 8 inches (1⁄16 of 10 by 16-inch melon, about 2 pounds with rind).[5]	925	93	115	2	1

[5]Measure and weight apply to entire vegetable or fruit including parts not usually eaten.

Fatty acids			Carbo-hy-drate	Cal-cium	Iron	Vita-min A value	Thia-min	Ribo-flavin	Niacin	Ascor-bic acid
Satu-rated (total)	Unsaturated									
	Oleic	Lin-oleic								
Grams	Grams	Grams	Grams	Milli-grams	Milli-grams	Inter-national units	Milli-grams	Milli-grams	Milli-grams	Milli-grams
------	------	------	18	14	1.1	440	.02	.04	.4	1
------	------	------	78	60	4.5	1,860	.08	.18	1.7	2
------	------	------	49	36	10.5	-------	.03	.03	1.0	[8] 5
------	------	------	11	9	.5	Trace	.02	.01	.1	Trace
------	------	------	128	102	5.8	30	.18	.13	.8	2
------	------	------	17	27	1.1	160	.04	.11	1.1	31
------	------	------	70	37	1.7	200	.06	.17	1.7	59
------	------	------	98	212	1.6	220	.06	.15	.7	17
------	------	------	13	31	1.5	90	.04	.10	1.0	88
------	------	------	79	40	2.0	90	.06	.17	1.5	150
------	------	------	10	34	.3	360	.05	.02	.1	27
------	------	------	30	45	.5	1,050	.15	.05	.2	55
------	------	------	27	30	2.1	2,510	.13	.13	.7	30

[8]This is the amount from the fruit. Additional ascorbic acid may be added by the manufacturer. Refer to the label for this information.

TABLE 1.—NUTRITIVE VALUES OF THE

GRAIN PRODUCTS

	Food, approximate measure, and weight (in grams)			Water	Food energy	Protein	Fat
			Grams	Per-cent	Calo-ries	Grams	Grams
	Bagel, 3-in. diam.:						
333	Egg_____	1 bagel_____	55	32	165	6	2
334	Water_____	1 bagel_____	55	29	165	6	2
335	Barley, pearled, light, uncooked.	1 cup_____	200	11	700	16	2
336	Biscuits, baking powder from home recipe with enriched flour, 2-in. diam.	1 biscuit_____	28	27	105	2	5
337	Biscuits, baking powder from mix, 2-in. diam.	1 biscuit_____	28	28	90	2	3
338	Bran flakes (40% bran), added thiamin and iron.	1 cup_____	35	3	105	4	1
339	Bran flakes with raisins, added thiamin and iron.	1 cup_____	50	7	145	4	1
	Breads:						
340	Boston brown bread, slice 3 by ¾ in.	1 slice_____	48	45	100	3	1
	Cracked-wheat bread:						
341	Loaf, 1 lb._____	1 loaf_____	454	35	1,190	40	10
342	Slice, 18 slices per loaf.	1 slice_____	25	35	65	2	1
	French or vienna bread:						
343	Enriched, 1 lb. loaf__	1 loaf_____	454	31	1,315	41	14
344	Unenriched, 1 lb. loaf.	1 loaf_____	454	31	1,315	41	14
	Italian bread:						
345	Enriched, 1 lb. loaf__	1 loaf_____	454	32	1,250	41	4
346	Unenriched, 1 lb. loaf.	1 loaf_____	454	32	1,250	41	4

EDIBLE PART OF FOODS (*continued*)

| Fatty acids | | | Carbo-hydrate | Cal-cium | Iron | Vita-min A value | Thia-min | Ribo-flavin | Niacin | Ascor-bic acid |
| Satu-rated (total) | Unsaturated | | | | | | | | | |
	Oleic	Lin-oleic								
Grams	*Grams*	*Grams*	*Grams*	*Milli-grams*	*Milli-grams*	*Inter-national units*	*Milli-grams*	*Milli-grams*	*Milli-grams*	*Milli-grams*
-----	-----	-----	28	9	1.2	30	0.14	0.10	1.2	0
-----	-----	-----	30	8	1.2	0	.15	.11	1.4	0
Trace	1	1	158	32	4.0	0	.24	.10	6.2	0
1	2	1	13	34	.4	Trace	.06	.06	.1	Trace
1	1	1	15	19	.6	Trace	.08	.07	.6	Trace
-----	-----	-----	28	25	12.3	0	.14	.06	2.2	0
-----	-----	-----	40	28	13.5	Trace	.16	.07	2.7	0
-----	-----	-----	22	43	.9	0	.05	.03	.6	0
2	5	2	236	399	5.0	Trace	.53	.41	5.9	Trace
-----	-----	-----	13	22	.3	Trace	.03	.02	.3	Trace
3	8	2	251	195	10.0	Trace	1.27	1.00	11.3	Trace
3	8	2	251	195	3.2	Trace	.36	.36	3.6	Trace
Trace	1	2	256	77	10.0	0	1.32	.91	11.8	0
Trace	1	2	256	77	3.2	0	.41	.27	3.6	0

TABLE 1.—NUTRITIVE VALUES OF THE

	Food, approximate measure, and weight (in grams)			Water	Food energy	Pro-tein	Fat
			Grams	Per-cent	Calo-ries	Grams	Grams
	GRAIN PRODUCTS—Continued						
	Bread—Continued						
	Raisin bread:						
347	Loaf, 1 lb_____	1 loaf_____	454	35	1,190	30	13
348	Slice, 18 slices per loaf.	1 slice_____	25	35	65	2	1
	Rye bread:						
	American, light (⅓ rye, ⅔ wheat):						
349	Loaf, 1 lb_____	1 loaf_____	454	36	1,100	41	5
350	Slice, 18 slices per loaf.	1 slice_____	25	36	60	2	Trace
351	Pumpernickel, loaf, 1 lb.	1 loaf_____	454	34	1,115	41	5
	White bread, enriched: [15]						
	Soft-crumb type:						
352	Loaf, 1 lb_____	1 loaf_____	454	36	1,225	39	15
353	Slice, 18 slices per loaf.	1 slice_____	25	36	70	2	1
354	Slice, toasted____	1 slice_____	22	25	70	2	1
355	Slice, 22 slices per loaf.	1 slice_____	20	36	55	2	1
356	Slice, toasted____	1 slice_____	17	25	55	2	1
357	Loaf, 1½ lbs_____	1 loaf_____	680	36	1,835	59	22
358	Slice, 24 slices per loaf.	1 slice_____	28	36	75	2	1
359	Slice, toasted____	1 slice_____	24	25	75	2	1
360	Slice, 28 slices per loaf.	1 slice_____	24	36	65	2	1
361	Slice, toasted____	1 slice_____	21	25	65	2	1
	Firm-crumb type:						
362	Loaf, 1 lb_____	1 loaf_____	454	35	1,245	41	17

[15]Values for iron, thiamin, riboflavin, and niacin per pound of unenriched white bread would be as follows:

EDIBLE PART OF FOODS (*continued*)

Fatty acids			Carbo-hy-drate	Cal-cium	Iron	Vita-min A value	Thia-min	Ribo-flavin	Niacin	Ascor-bic acid
Satu-rated (total)	Unsaturated									
	Oleic	Lin-oleic								
Grams	Grams	Grams	Grams	Milli-grams	Milli-grams	Inter-national units	Milli-grams	Milli-grams	Milli-grams	Milli-grams
3	8	2	243	322	5.9	Trace	.23	.41	3.2	Trace
------	------	------	13	18	.3	Trace	.01	.02	.2	Trace
------	------	------	236	340	7.3	0	.82	.32	6.4	0
------	------	------	13	19	.4	0	.05	.02	.4	0
			241	381	10.9	0	1.04	.64	5.4	0
3	8	2	229	381	11.3	Trace	1.13	.95	10.9	Trace
------	------	------	13	21	.6	Trace	.06	.05	.6	Trace
------	------	------	13	21	.6	Trace	.06	.05	.6	Trace
------	------	------	10	17	.5	Trace	.05	.04	.5	Trace
------	------	------	10	17	.5	Trace	.05	.04	.5	Trace
5	12	3	343	571	17.0	Trace	1.70	1.43	16.3	Trace
------	------	------	14	24	.7	Trace	.07	.06	.7	Trace
------	------	------	14	24	.7	Trace	.07	.06	.7	Trace
------	------	------	12	20	.6	Trace	.06	.05	.6	Trace
------	------	------	12	20	.6	Trace	.06	.05	.6	Trace
4	10	2	228	435	11.3	Trace	1.22	.91	10.9	Trace

	Iron Milligrams	Thiamin Milligrams	Riboflavin Milligrams	Niacin Milligrams
Soft crumb	3.2	.31	.39	5.0
Firm crumb	3.2	.32	.59	4.1

TABLE 1.—NUTRITIVE VALUES OF THE

	Food, approximate measure, and weight (in grams)		Water	Food energy	Pro-tein	Fat
	GRAIN PRODUCTS—Continued					
	Bread—Continued					
	Firm-crumb type—Continued	*Grams*	*Per-cent*	*Calo-ries*	*Grams*	*Grams*
363	Slice, 20 slices per loaf.	1 slice_____ 23	35	65	2	1
364	Slice, toasted____	1 slice_____ 20	24	65	2	1
365	Loaf, 2 lbs._____	1 loaf_____ 907	35	2,495	82	34
366	Slice, 34 slices per loaf.	1 slice_____ 27	35	75	2	1
367	Slice, toasted____	1 slice_____ 23	35	75	2	1
	Whole-wheat bread, soft-crumb type:					
368	Loaf, 1 lb._____	1 loaf_____ 454	36	1,095	41	12
369	Slice, 16 slices per loaf.	1 slice_____ 28	36	65	3	1
370	Slice, toasted_____	1 slice_____ 24	24	65	3	1
	Whole-wheat bread, firm-crumb type:					
371	Loaf, 1 lb._____	1 loaf_____ 454	36	1,100	48	14
372	Slice, 18 slices per loaf.	1 slice_____ 25	36	60	3	1
373	Slice, toasted_____	1 slice_____ 21	24	60	3	1
374	Breadcrumbs, dry, grated_	1 cup_____ 100	6	390	13	5
375	Buckwheat flour, light, sifted.	1 cup_____ 98	12	340	6	1
376	Bulgur, canned, seasoned_	1 cup_____ 135	56	245	8	4
	Cakes made from cake mixes:					
	Angelfood:					
377	Whole cake_____	1 cake_____ 635	34	1,645	36	1
378	Piece, 1/12 of 10-in. diam. cake.	1 piece_____ 53	34	135	3	Trace
	Cupcakes, small, 2 1/2 in. diam.:					
379	Without icing_____	1 cupcake___ 25	26	90	1	3
380	With chocolate icing_	1 cupcake___ 36	22	130	2	5

EDIBLE PART OF FOODS (*continued*)

Fatty acids			Carbo-hy-drate	Cal-cium	Iron	Vita-min A value	Thia-min	Ribo-flavin	Niacin	Ascor-bic acid
Satu-rated (total)	Unsaturated									
	Oleic	Lin-oleic								
Grams	*Grams*	*Grams*	*Grams*	*Milli-grams*	*Milli-grams*	*Inter-national units*	*Milli-grams*	*Milli-grams*	*Milli-grams*	*Milli-grams*
------	------	------	12	22	.6	Trace	.06	.05	.6	Trace
------	------	------	12	22	.6	Trace	.06	.05	.6	Trace
8	20	4	455	871	22.7	Trace	2.45	1.81	21.8	Trace
------	------	------	14	26	.7	Trace	.07	.05	.6	Trace
------	------	------	14	26	.7	Trace	.07	.05	.6	Trace
2	6	2	224	381	13.6	Trace	1.36	.45	12.7	Trace
------	------	------	14	24	.8	Trace	.09	.03	.8	Trace
------	------	------	14	24	.8	Trace	.09	.03	.8	Trace
3	6	3	216	449	13.6	Trace	1.18	0.54	12.7	Trace
------	------	------	12	25	.8	Trace	.06	.03	.7	Trace
------	------	------	12	25	.8	Trace	.06	.03	.7	Trace
1	2	1	73	122	3.6	Trace	.22	.30	3.5	Trace
------	------	------	78	11	1.0	0	.08	.04	.4	0
------	------	------	44	27	1.9	0	.08	.05	4.1	0
------	------	------	377	603	1.9	0	.03	.70	.6	0
------	------	------	32	50	.2	0	Trace	.06	.1	0
1	1	1	14	40	.1	40	.01	.03	.1	Trace
2	2	1	21	47	.3	60	.01	.04	.1	Trace

TABLE 1.—NUTRITIVE VALUES OF THE

	Food, approximate measure, and weight (in grams)	Water	Food energy	Pro-tein	Fat
	GRAIN PRODUCTS—Continued				
	Cakes made from cake mixes—Con. *Grams*	*Per-cent*	*Calo-ries*	*Grams*	*Grams*
	Devil's food, 2-layer, with chocolate icing:				
381	Whole cake_____ 1 cake_____1,107	24	3,755	49	136
382	Piece, ⅟₁₆ of 9-in. 1 piece_____ 69	24	235	3	9
	diam. cake.				
383	Cupcake, small, 2½ 1 cupcake___ 35	24	120	2	4
	in. diam.				
	Gingerbread:				
384	Whole cake_____ 1 cake_____ 570	37	1,575	18	39
385	Piece, ⅑ of 8-in. 1 piece_____ 63	37	175	2	4
	square cake.				
	White, 2-layer, with chocolate icing:				
386	Whole cake_____ 1 cake_____1,140	21	4,000	45	122
387	Piece, ⅟₁₆ of 9-in. 1 piece_____ 71	21	250	3	8
	diam. cake.				
	Cakes made from home recipes: [16]				
388	Boston cream pie; 1 piece_____ 69	35	210	4	6
	piece ⅟₁₂ of 8-in. diam.				
	Fruitcake, dark, made with enriched flour:				
389	Loaf, 1-lb._____ 1 loaf_____ 454	18	1,720	22	69
390	Slice, 1/30 of 8-in. 1 slice_____ 15	18	55	1	2
	loaf.				
	Plain sheet cake:				
	Without icing:				
391	Whole cake_____ 1 cake_____ 777	25	2,830	35	108
392	Piece, ⅑ of 9-in. 1 piece_____ 86	25	315	4	12
	square cake.				
393	With boiled white 1 piece_____ 114	23	400	4	12
	icing, piece, ⅑ of 9-in. square cake.				

[16]Unenriched cake flour used unless otherwise specified.

EDIBLE PART OF FOODS (continued)

Fatty acids			Carbo-hy-drate	Cal-cium	Iron	Vita-min A value	Thia-min	Ribo-flavin	Niacin	Ascor-bic acid
Satu-rated (total)	Unsaturated									
	Oleic	Lin-oleic								
Grams	Grams	Grams	Grams	Milli-grams	Milli-grams	Inter-national units	Milli-grams	Milli-grams	Milli-grams	Milli-grams
54	58	16	645	653	8.9	1,660	.33	.89	3.3	1
3	4	1	40	41	.6	100	.02	.06	.2	Trace
1	2	Trace	20	21	.3	50	.01	.03	.1	Trace
10	19	9	291	513	9.1	Trace	.17	.51	4.6	2
1	2	1	32	57	1.0	Trace	.02	.06	.5	Trace
45	54	17	716	1,129	5.7	680	.23	.91	2.3	2
3	3	1	45	70	.4	40	.01	.06	.1	Trace
2	3	1	34	46	.3	140	.02	.08	.1	Trace
15	37	13	271	327	11.8	540	.59	.64	3.6	2
Trace	1	Trace	9	11	.4	20	.02	.02	.1	Trace
30	52	21	434	497	3.1	1,320	.16	.70	1.6	2
3	6	2	48	55	.3	150	.02	.08	.2	Trace
3	6	2	71	56	.3	150	.02	.08	.2	Trace

TABLE 1.—NUTRITIVE VALUES OF THE

	Food, approximate measure, and weight (in grams)		Water	Food energy	Pro-tein	Fat

GRAIN PRODUCTS—Continued

		Grams	Per-cent	Calo-ries	Grams	Grams
	Cakes made from home recipes —Con.					
	Pound:					
394	Loaf, 8½ by 3½ by 3in.	1 loaf_____ 514	17	2,430	29	152
395	Slice, ½-in. thick____	1 slice_____ 30	17	140	2	9
	Sponge:					
396	Whole cake_____	1 cake_____ 790	32	2,345	60	45
397	Piece, ¹⁄₁₂ of 10-in. diam. cake.	1 piece_____ 66	32	195	5	4
	Yellow, 2-layer, without icing:					
398	Whole cake_____	1 cake_____ 870	24	3,160	39	111
399	Piece, ¹⁄₁₆ of 9-in. diam. cake.	1 piece_____ 54	24	200	2	7
	Yellow, 2-layer, with chocolate icing:					
400	Whole cake_____	1 cake_____1,203	21	4,390	51	156
401	Piece, ¹⁄₁₆ of 9-in. diam. cake.	1 piece_____ 75	21	275	3	10
	Cake icings. See Sugars, Sweets.					
	Cookies:					
	Brownies with nuts:					
402	Made from home recipe with en-riched flour.	1 brownie____ 20	10	95	1	6
403	Made from mix_____	1 brownie____ 20	11	85	1	4
	Chocolate chip:					
404	Made from home recipe with en-riched flour.	1 cookie_____ 10	3	50	1	3
405	Commercial_____	1 cookie_____ 10	3	50	1	2

EDIBLE PART OF FOODS *(continued)*

Fatty acids			Carbo-hy-drate	Cal-cium	Iron	Vita-min A value	Thia-min	Ribo-flavin	Niacin	Ascor-bic acid
Satu-rated (total)	Unsaturated									
	Oleic	Lin-oleic								
Grams	*Grams*	*Grams*	*Grams*	*Milli-grams*	*Milli-grams*	*Inter-national units*	*Milli-grams*	*Milli-grams*	*Milli-grams*	*Milli-grams*
34	68	17	242	108	4.1	1,440	.15	.46	1.0	0
2	4	1	14	6	.2	80	.01	.03	.1	0
14	20	4	427	237	9.5	3,560	.40	1.11	1.6	Trace
1	2	Trace	36	20	.8	300	.03	.09	.1	Trace
31	53	22	506	618	3.5	1,310	.17	.70	1.7	2
2	3	1	32	39	.2	80	.01	.04	.1	Trace
55	69	23	727	818	7.2	1,920	.24	.96	2.4	Trace
3	4	1	45	51	.5	120	.02	.06	.2	Trace
1	3	1	10	8	.4	40	.04	.02	.1	Trace
1	2	1	13	9	.4	20	.03	.02	.1	Trace
1	1	1	6	4	0.2	10	0.01	0.01	0.1	Trace
1	1	Trace	7	4	.2	10	Trace	Trace	Trace	Trace

TABLE 1.—NUTRITIVE VALUES OF THE

	Food, approximate measure, and weight (in grams)		Grams	Water Per-cent	Food energy Calo-ries	Pro-tein Grams	Fat Grams
	GRAIN PRODUCTS—Continued						
	Cookies—Continued						
406	Fig bars, commercial___	1 cookie_____	14	14	50	1	1
407	Sandwich, chocolate or vanilla, commercial.	1 cookie_____	10	2	50	1	2
	Corn flakes, added nutrients:						
408	Plain_____	1 cup_____	25	4	100	2	Trace
409	Sugar-covered_____	1 cup_____	40	2	155	2	Trace
	Corn (hominy) grits, degermed, cooked:						
410	Enriched_____	1 cup_____	245	87	125	3	Trace
411	Unenriched_____	1 cup_____	245	87	125	3	Trace
	Cornmeal:						
412	Whole-ground, unbolted, dry.	1 cup_____	122	12	435	11	5
413	Bolted (nearly whole-grain) dry.	1 cup_____	122	12	440	11	4
	Degermed, enriched:						
414	Dry form_____	1 cup_____	138	12	500	11	2
415	Cooked_____	1 cup_____	240	88	120	3	1
	Degermed, unenriched:						
416	Dry form_____	1 cup_____	138	12	500	11	2
417	Cooked_____	1 cup_____	240	88	120	3	1
418	Corn muffins, made with enriched de-germed cornmeal and enriched flour; muffin 2⅜-in. diam.	1 muffin ____	40	33	125	3	4
419	Corn muffins, made with mix, egg, and milk; muffin 2⅜-in. diam.	1 muffin_____	40	30	130	3	4
420	Corn, puffed, presweet-ened, added nutrients.	1 cup_____	30	2	115	1	Trace

[17]This value is based on product made from yellow varieties of corn; white varieties contain only a trace.

EDIBLE PART OF FOODS (*continued*)

Fatty acids			Carbohydrate	Calcium	Iron	Vitamin A value	Thiamin	Riboflavin	Niacin	Ascorbic acid
Saturated (total)	Unsaturated									
	Oleic	Linoleic								
Grams	*Grams*	*Grams*	*Grams*	*Milligrams*	*Milligrams*	*International units*	*Milligrams*	*Milligrams*	*Milligrams*	*Milligrams*
------	------	------	11	11	.2	20	Trace	.01	.1	Trace
1	1	Trace	7	2	.1	0	Trace	Trace	.1	0
------	------	------	21	4	.4	0	.11	.02	.5	0
------	------	------	36	5	.4	0	.16	.02	.8	0
------	------	------	27	2	.7	[17] 150	.10	.07	1.0	0
------	------	------	27	2	.2	[17] 150	.05	.02	.5	0
1	2	2	90	24	2.9	[17] 620	.46	.13	2.4	0
Trace	1	2	91	21	2.2	[17] 590	.37	.10	2.3	0
------	------	------	108	8	4.0	[17] 610	.61	.36	4.8	0
------	------	------	26	2	1.0	[17] 140	.14	.10	1.2	0
------	------	------	108	8	1.5	[17] 610	.19	.07	1.4	0
------	------	------	26	2	.5	[17] 140	.05	.02	.2	0
2	2	Trace	19	42	.7	[17] 120	.08	.09	.6	Trace
1	2	1	20	96	.6	100	.07	.08	.6	Trace
------	------	------	27	3	.5	0	.13	.05	.6	0

TABLE 1.—NUTRITIVE VALUES OF THE

	Food, approximate measure, and weight (in grams)			Water	Food energy	Protein	Fat
	GRAIN PRODUCTS						
			Grams	*Per-cent*	*Calo-ries*	*Grams*	*Grams*
421	Corn, shredded, added nutrients.	1 cup	25	3	100	2	Trace
	Crackers:						
422	Graham, 2½-in. square	4 crackers	28	6	110	2	3
423	Saltines	4 crackers	11	4	50	1	1
	Danish pastry, plain (without fruit or nuts):						
424	Packaged ring, 12 ounces.	1 ring	340	22	1,435	25	80
425	Round piece, approx. 4¼-in. diam. by 1 in.	1 pastry	65	22	275	5	15
426	Ounce	1 oz.	28	22	120	2	7
427	Doughnuts, cake type	1 doughnut	32	24	125	1	6
428	Farina, quick-cooking, enriched, cooked.	1 cup	245	89	105	3	Trace
	Macaroni, cooked:						
	Enriched:						
429	Cooked, firm stage (undergoes additional cooking in a food mixture).	1 cup	130	64	190	6	1
430	Cooked until tender	1 cup	140	72	155	5	1
	Unenriched:						
431	Cooked, firm stage (undergoes additional cooking in a food mixture).	1 cup	130	64	190	6	1
432	Cooked until tender	1 cup	140	72	155	5	1
433	Macaroni (enriched) and cheese, baked.	1 cup	200	58	430	17	22
434	Canned	1 cup	240	80	230	9	10

[18]Based on product made with enriched flour. With enriched flour, approximate values per doughnut are: Iron, 0.2 milligram; thiamin, 0.01 milligram; riboflavin, 0.03 milligram; niacin, 0.2 milligram.

EDIBLE PART OF FOODS *(continued)*

Fatty acids			Carbo-hy-drate	Cal-cium	Iron	Vita-min A value	Thia-min	Ribo-flavin	Niacin	Ascor-bic acid
Satu-rated (total)	Unsaturated									
	Oleic	Lin-oleic								
Grams	*Grams*	*Grams*	*Grams*	*Milli-grams*	*Milli-grams*	*Inter-national units*	*Milli-grams*	*Milli-grams*	*Milli-grams*	*Milli-grams*
------	------	------	22	1	.6	0	.11	.05	.5	0
------	------	------	21	11	.4	0	.01	.06	.4	0
------	1	------	8	2	.1	0	Trace	Trace	.1	0
24	37	15	155	170	3.1	1,050	.24	.51	2.7	Trace
5	7	3	30	33	.6	200	.05	.10	.5	Trace
2	3	1	13	14	.3	90	.02	.04	.2	Trace
1	4	Trace	16	13	[18].4	30	[18].05	[18].05	[18].4	Trace
------	------	------	22	147	[19].7	0	[19].12	[19].07	[19]1.0	0
------	------	------	39	14	[19]1.4	0	[19].23	[19].14	[19]1.8	0
------	------	------	32	8	[19]1.3	0	[19].20	[19].11	[19]1.5	0
------	------	------	39	14	.7	0	.03	.03	.5	0
------	------	------	32	11	.6	0	.01	.01	.4	0
10	9	2	40	362	1.8	860	.20	.40	1.8	Trace
4	3	1	26	199	1.0	260	.12	.24	1.0	Trace

[19]Iron, thiamin, riboflavin, and niacin are based on the minimum levels of enrichment specified in standards of identity promulgated under the Federal Food, Drug, and Cosmetic Act.

TABLE 1.—NUTRITIVE VALUES OF THE

Food, approximate measure, and weight (in grams)		Water	Food energy	Pro-tein	Fat
GRAIN PRODUCTS—Continued					
	Grams	Per-cent	Calo-ries	Grams	Grams
435 Muffins, with enriched white flour; muffin, 3-inch diam.	1 muffin ____ 40	38	120	3	4
Noodles (egg noodles), cooked:					
436 Enriched_____	1 cup_____ 160	70	200	7	2
437 Unenriched_____	1 cup_____ 160	70	200	7	2
438 Oats (with or without corn) puffed, added nutrients.	1 cup_____ 25	3	100	3	1
439 Oatmeal or rolled oats, cooked.	1 cup_____ 240	87	130	5	2
Pancakes, 4-inch diam.:					
440 Wheat, enriched flour (home recipe).	1 cake_____ 27	50	60	2	2
441 Buckwheat (made from mix with egg and milk).	1 cake_____ 27	58	55	2	2
442 Plain or buttermilk (made from mix with egg and milk).	1 cake_____ 27	51	60	2	2
Pie (piecrust made with unenriched flour):					
Sector, 4-in., ⅐ of 9-in. diam. pie:					
443 Apple (2-crust)_____	1 sector_____ 135	48	350	3	15
444 Butterscotch (1-crust)__	1 sector_____ 130	45	350	6	14
445 Cherry (2-crust)_____	1 sector_____ 135	47	350	4	15
446 Custard (1-crust)_____	1 sector_____ 130	58	285	8	14
447 Lemon meringue (1-crust).	1 sector_____ 120	47	305	4	12
448 Mince (2-crust)_____	1 sector_____ 135	43	365	3	16
449 Pecan (1-crust)_____	1 sector_____ 118	20	490	6	27

[19]Iron, thiamin, riboflavin, and niacin are based on the minimum levels of enrichment specified in standards of identity promulgated under the Federal Food, Drug, and Cosmetic Act.

Fatty acids			Carbo-hydrate	Cal-cium	Iron	Vita-min A value	Thia-min	Ribo-flavin	Niacin	Ascor-bic acid
Satu-rated (total)	Unsaturated									
	Oleic	Lin-oleic								
Grams	Grams	Grams	Grams	Milli-grams	Milli-grams	Inter-national units	Milli-grams	Milli-grams	Milli-grams	Milli-grams
1	2	1	17	42	.6	40	.07	.09	.6	Trace
1	1	Trace	37	16	[19]1.4	110	[19].22	[19].13	[19]1.9	0
1	1	Trace	37	16	1.0	110	.05	.03	.6	0
------	------	------	19	44	1.2	0	0.24	0.04	0.5	0
------	------	1	23	22	1.4	0	.19	.05	.2	0
Trace	1	Trace	9	27	.4	30	.05	.06	.4	Trace
1	1	Trace	6	59	.4	60	.03	.04	.2	Trace
1	1	Trace	9	58	.3	70	.04	.06	.2	Trace
4	7	3	51	11	.4	40	.03	.03	.5	1
5	6	2	50	98	1.2	340	.04	.13	.3	Trace
4	7	3	52	19	.4	590	.03	.03	.7	Trace
5	6	2	30	125	.8	300	.07	.21	.4	0
4	6	2	45	17	.6	200	.04	.10	.2	4
4	8	3	56	38	1.4	Trace	.09	.05	.5	1
4	16	5	60	55	3.3	190	.19	.08	.4	Trace

TABLE 1.—NUTRITIVE VALUES OF THE

	Food, approximate measure, and weight (in grams)			Water	Food energy	Pro-tein	Fat

GRAIN PRODUCTS—Continued

				Per-cent	*Calo-ries*	*Grams*	*Grams*
	Pie (piecrust made with unenriched flour) *Grams*						
450	Pineapple chiffon (1-crust).	1 sector_____	93	41	265	6	11
451	Pumpkin (1-crust)_____	1 sector_____	130	59	275	5	15
	Piecrust, baked shell for pie made with:						
452	Enriched flour_____	1 shell_____	180	15	900	11	60
453	Unenriched flour_____	1 shell_____	180	15	900	11	60
	Piecrust mix including stick form:						
454	Package, 10-oz., for double crust.	1 pkg_____	284	9	1,480	20	93
455	Pizza (cheese) 5½-in. sector; ⅛ of 14-in. diam. pie.	1 sector_____	75	45	185	7	6
	Popcorn, popped:						
456	Plain, large kernel_____	1 cup_____	6	4	25	1	Trace
457	With oil and salt_____	1 cup_____	9	3	40	1	2
458	Sugar coated_____	1 cup_____	35	4	135	2	1
	Pretzels:						
459	Dutch, twisted_____	1 pretzel____	16	5	60	2	1
460	Thin, twisted_____	1 pretzel____	6	5	25	1	Trace
461	Stick, small, 2¼ inches_	10 sticks____	3	5	10	Trace	Trace
462	Stick, regular, 3⅛ inches.	5 sticks_____	3	5	10	Trace	Trace
	Rice, white:						
	Enriched:						
463	Raw_____	1 cup_____	185	12	670	12	1
464	Cooked_____	1 cup_____	205	73	225	4	Trace
465	Instant, ready-to-serve.	1 cup_____	165	73	180	4	Trace
466	Unenriched, cooked____	1 cup_____	205	73	225	4	Trace
467	Parboiled, cooked_____	1 cup_____	175	73	185	4	Trace

[20]Iron, thiamin, and niacin are based on the minimum levels of enrichment specified in standards of identity promulgated under the Federal Food, Drug, and Cosmetic Act. Riboflavin is based on unenriched rice. When the minimum level of enrichment

EDIBLE PART OF FOODS (continued)

Fatty acids			Carbo-hy-drate	Cal-cium	Iron	Vita-min A value	Thia-min	Ribo-flavin	Niacin	Ascor-bic acid
Satu-rated (total)	Unsaturated									
	Oleic	Lin-oleic								
Grams	Grams	Grams	Grams	Milli-grams	Milli-grams	Inter-national units	Milli-grams	Milli-grams	Milli-grams	Milli-grams
3	5	2	36	22	.8	320	.04	.08	.4	1
5	6	2	32	66	.7	3,210	.04	.13	.7	Trace
16	28	12	79	25	3.1	0	.36	.25	3.2	0
16	28	12	79	25	.9	0	.05	.05	.9	0
23	46	21	141	131	1.4	0	.11	.11	2.0	0
2	3	Trace	27	107	.7	290	.04	.12	.7	4
------	------	------	5	1	.2	------	------	.01	.1	0
1	Trace	Trace	5	1	.2	------	------	.01	.2	0
------	------	------	30	2	.5	------	------	.02	.4	0
------	------	------	12	4	.2	0	Trace	Trace	.1	0
------	------	------	5	1	.1	0	Trace	Trace	Trace	0
------	------	------	2	1	Trace	0	Trace	Trace	Trace	0
------	------	------	2	1	Trace	0	Trace	Trace	Trace	0
------	------	------	149	44	[20]5.4	0	[20].81	[20].06	[20]6.5	0
------	------	------	50	21	[20]1.8	0	[20].23	[20].02	[20]2.1	0
------	------	------	40	5	[20]1.3	0	[20].21	[20]---	[20]1.7	0
------	------	------	50	21	.4	0	.04	.02	.8	0
------	------	------	41	33	[20]1.4	0	[20].19	[20]---	[20]2.1	0

for riboflavin specified in the standards of identity becomes effective the value will be 0.12 milligram per cup of parboiled rice and of white rice.

TABLE 1.—NUTRITIVE VALUES OF THE

	Food, approximate measure, and weight (in grams)			Water	Food energy	Pro-tein	Fat

GRAIN PRODUCTS—Continued

			Grams	Per-cent	Calo-ries	Grams	Grams
468	Rice, puffed, added nutrients.	1 cup	15	4	60	1	Trace
	Rolls, enriched:						
	Cloverleaf or pan:						
469	Home recipe	1 roll	35	26	120	3	3
470	Commercial	1 roll	28	31	85	2	2
471	Frankfurter or hamburger.	1 roll	40	31	120	3	2
472	Hard, round or rectangular.	1 roll	50	25	155	5	2
473	Rye wafers, whole-grain, 1 ⅞ by 3 ½ inches.	2 wafers	13	6	45	2	Trace
474	Spaghetti, cooked, tender stage, enriched.	1 cup	140	72	155	5	1
	Spaghetti with meat balls, and tomato sauce:						
475	Home recipe	1 cup	248	70	330	19	12
476	Canned	1 cup	250	78	260	12	10
	Spaghetti in tomato sauce with cheese:						
477	Home recipe	1 cup	250	77	260	9	9
478	Canned	1 cup	250	80	190	6	2
479	Waffles, with enriched flour, 7-in. diam.	1 waffle	75	41	210	7	7
480	Waffles, made from mix, enriched, egg and milk added, 7-in. diam.	1 waffle	75	42	205	7	8
481	Wheat, puffed, added nutrients.	1 cup	15	3	55	2	Trace
482	Wheat, shredded, plain	1 biscuit	25	7	90	2	1
483	Wheat flakes, added nutrients.	1 cup	30	4	105	3	Trace

[19]Iron, thiamin, riboflavin, and niacin are based on the minimum levels of enrichment specified in standards of identity promulgated under the Federal Food, Drug, and Cosmetic Act.

Saturated (total)	Unsaturated		Carbohydrate	Calcium	Iron	Vitamin A value	Thiamin	Riboflavin	Niacin	Ascorbic acid
Fatty acids										
	Oleic	Linoleic								
Grams	Grams	Grams	Grams	Milligrams	Milligrams	International units	Milligrams	Milligrams	Milligrams	Milligrams
-----	-----	-----	13	3	.3	0	.07	.01	.7	0
1	1	1	20	16	.7	30	.09	.09	.8	Trace
Trace	1	Trace	15	21	.5	Trace	.08	.05	.6	Trace
1	1	1	21	30	.8	Trace	.11	.07	.9	Trace
Trace	1	Trace	30	24	1.2	Trace	.13	.12	1.4	Trace
-----	-----	-----	10	7	.5	0	.04	.03	.2	0
-----	-----	-----	32	11	[19]1.3	0	[19].20	[19].11	[19]1.5	0
4	6	1	39	124	3.7	1,590	0.25	0.30	4.0	22
2	3	4	28	53	3.3	1,000	.15	.18	2.3	5
2	5	1	37	80	2.3	1,080	.25	.18	2.3	13
1	1	1	38	40	2.8	930	.35	.28	4.5	10
2	4	1	28	85	1.3	250	.13	.19	1.0	Trace
3	3	1	27	179	1.0	170	.11	.17	.7	Trace
-----	-----	-----	12	4	.6	0	.08	.03	1.2	0
-----	-----	-----	20	11	.9	0	.06	.03	1.1	0
-----	-----	-----	24	12	1.3	0	.19	.04	1.5	0

TABLE 1.—NUTRITIVE VALUES OF THE

Food, approximate measure, and weight (in grams)		Water	Food energy	Pro-tein	Fat
GRAIN PRODUCTS—Continued					
Cakes made from home recipes —Con.	*Grams*	*Per-cent*	*Calo-ries*	*Grams*	*Grams*
Wheat flours:					
484	Whole-wheat, from hard wheats, stirred.	1 cup_____	120	12	400	16	2
	All-purpose or family flour, enriched:					
485	Sifted_____ 1 cup_____	115	12	420	12	1
486	Unsifted_____ 1 cup_____	125	12	455	13	1
487	Self-rising, enriched____ 1 cup_____	125	12	440	12	1
488	Cake or pastry flour, 1 cup_____ sifted.	96	12	350	7	1
	FATS, OILS					
	Butter:					
	Regular, 4 sticks per pound:					
489	Stick_____ ½ cup_____	113	16	810	1	92
490	Tablespoon (approx. 1 tbsp._____ ⅛ stick).	14	16	100	Trace	12
491	Pat (1-in. sq. ⅓-in. 1 pat_____ high; 90 per lb.).	5	16	35	Trace	4
	Whipped, 6 sticks or 2, 8-oz. containers per pound:					
492	Stick_____ ½ cup_____	76	16	540	1	61
493	Tablespoon (approx. 1 tbsp._____ ⅛ stick).	9	16	65	Trace	8
494	Pat (1¼-in. sq. ⅓-in. 1 pat_____ high; 120 per lb.).	4	16	25	Trace	3
	Fats, cooking:					
495	Lard_____ 1 cup_____	205	0	1,850	0	205
496	1 tbsp._____	13	0	115	0	13
497	Vegetable fats_____ 1 cup_____	200	0	1,770	0	200
498	1 tbsp._____	13	0	110	0	13

[19]Iron, thiamin, riboflavin, and niacin are based on the minimum levels of enrich-ment specified in standards of identity promulgated under the Federal Food, Drug, and Cosmetic Act.

EDIBLE PART OF FOODS *(continued)*

Fatty acids			Carbo-hydrate	Cal-cium	Iron	Vita-min A value	Thia-min	Ribo-flavin	Niacin	Ascor-bic acid
Satu-rated (total)	Unsaturated									
	Oleic	Lin-oleic								
Grams	Grams	Grams	Grams	Milli-grams	Milli-grams	Inter-national units	Milli-grams	Milli-grams	Milli-grams	Milli-grams
Trace	1	1	85	49	4.0	0	.66	.14	5.2	0
-----	-----	-----	88	18	[19]3.3	0	[19].51	[19].30	[19]4.0	0
-----	-----	-----	95	20	[19]3.6	0	[19].55	[19].33	[19]4.4	0
-----	-----	-----	93	331	[19]3.6	0	[19].55	[19].33	[19]4.4	0
-----	-----	-----	76	16	.5	0	.03	.03	.7	0
51	30	3	1	23	0	[21]3,750	-----	-----	-----	0
6	4	Trace	Trace	3	0	[21]470	-----	-----	-----	0
2	1	Trace	Trace	1	0	[21]170	-----	-----	-----	0
34	20	2	Trace	15	0	[21]2,500	-----	-----	-----	0
4	3	Trace	Trace	2	0	[21]310	-----	-----	-----	0
2	1	Trace	Trace	1	0	[21]130	-----	-----	-----	0
78	94	20	0	0	0	0	0	0	0	0
5	6	1	0	0	0	0	0	0	0	0
50	100	44	0	0	0	-------	0	0	0	0
3	6	3	0	0	0	-------	0	0	0	0

[21]Year-round average.

TABLE 1.—NUTRITIVE VALUES OF THE

	Food, approximate measure, and weight (in grams)			Water	Food energy	Protein	Fat
	FATS, OILS—Continued						
			Grams	Percent	Calories	Grams	Grams
	Margarine:						
	Regular, 4 sticks per pound:						
499	Stick	½ cup	113	16	815	1	92
500	Tablespoon (approx. ⅛ stick).	1 tbsp.	14	16	100	Trace	12
501	Pat (1-in. sq. ⅓-in. high; 90 per lb.).	1 pat	5	16	35	Trace	4
	Whipped, 6 sticks per pound:						
502	Stick	½ cup	76	16	545	1	61
	Soft, 2 8-oz. tubs per pound:						
503	Tub	1 tub	227	16	1,635	1	184
504	Tablespoon	1 tbsp.	14	16	100	Trace	11
	Oils, salad or cooking:						
505	Corn	1 cup	220	0	1,945	0	220
506		1 tbsp.	14	0	125	0	14
507	Cottonseed	1 cup	220	0	1,945	0	220
508		1 tbsp.	14	0	125	0	14
509	Olive	1 cup	220	0	1,945	0	220
510		1 tbsp.	14	0	125	0	14
511	Peanut	1 cup	220	0	1,945	0	220
512		1 tbsp.	14	0	125	0	14
513	Safflower	1 cup	220	0	1,945	0	220
514		1 tbsp.	14	0	125	0	14
515	Soybean	1 cup	220	0	1,945	0	220
516		1 tbsp.	14	0	125	0	14
	Salad dressings:						
517	Blue cheese	1 tbsp.	15	32	75	1	8
	Commercial, mayonnaise type:						
518	Regular	1 tbsp.	15	41	65	Trace	6
519	Special dietary, low-calorie.	1 tbsp.	16	81	20	Trace	2

[22]Based on the average vitamin A content of fortified margarine. Federal specifications for fortified margarine require a minimum of 15,000 I.U. of vitamin A per pound.

EDIBLE PART OF FOODS *(continued)*

Fatty acids			Carbo-hydrate	Cal-cium	Iron	Vita-min A value	Thia-min	Ribo-flavin	Niacin	Ascor-bic acid
Satu-rated (total)	Unsaturated									
	Oleic	Lin-oleic								
Grams	Grams	Grams	Grams	Milli-grams	Milli-grams	Inter-national units	Milli-grams	Milli-grams	Milli-grams	Milli-grams
17	46	25	1	23	0	[22]3,750	------	------	------	0
2	6	3	Trace	3	0	[22]470	------	------	------	0
1	2	1	Trace	1	0	[22]170	------	------	------	0
11	31	17	Trace	15	0	[22]2,500	------	------	------	0
34	68	68	1	45	0	[22]7,500	------	------	------	0
2	4	4	Trace	3	0	[22]470	------	------	------	0
22	62	117	0	0	0	-------	0	0	0	0
1	4	7	0	0	0	-------	0	0	0	0
55	46	110	0	0	0	-------	0	0	0	0
4	3	7	0	0	0	-------	0	0	0	0
24	167	15	0	0	0	-------	0	0	0	0
2	11	1	0	0	0	-------	0	0	0	0
40	103	64	0	0	0	-------	0	0	0	0
3	7	4	0	0	0	-------	0	0	0	0
18	37	165	0	0	0	-------	0	0	0	0
1	2	10	0	0	0	-------	0	0	0	0
33	44	114	0	0	0	-------	0	0	0	0
2	3	7	0	0	0	-------	0	0	0	0
2	2	4	1	12	Trace	30	Trace	0.02	Trace	Trace
1	1	3	2	2	Trace	30	Trace	Trace	Trace	------
Trace	Trace	1	1	3	Trace	40	Trace	Trace	Trace	------

TABLE 1.—NUTRITIVE VALUES OF THE

	Food, approximate measure, and weight (in grams)			Water	Food energy	Pro-tein	Fat

FATS, OILS—Continued

	Salad dressings—Continued		Grams	Per-cent	Calo-ries	Grams	Grams
	French:						
520	Regular_____	1 tbsp._____	16	39	65	Trace	6
521	Special dietary, low-fat with artificial sweeteners.	1 tbsp._____	15	95	Trace	Trace	Trace
522	Home cooked, boiled_____	1 tbsp._____	16	68	25	1	2
523	Mayonnaise_____	1 tbsp._____	14	15	100	Trace	11
524	Thousand island_____	1 tbsp._____	16	32	80	Trace	8

SUGARS, SWEETS

	Cake icings:						
525	Chocolate made with milk and table fat.	1 cup_____	275	14	1,035	9	38
526	Coconut (with boiled icing).	1 cup_____	166	15	605	3	13
527	Creamy fudge from mix with water only.	1 cup_____	245	15	830	7	16
528	White, boiled_____	1 cup_____	94	18	300	1	0
	Candy:						
529	Caramels, plain or chocolate.	1 oz._____	28	8	115	1	3
530	Chocolate, milk, plain__	1 oz._____	28	1	145	2	9
531	Chocolate-coated peanuts.	1 oz._____	28	1	160	5	12
532	Fondant; mints, un-coated; candy corn.	1 oz._____	28	8	105	Trace	1
533	Fudge, plain_____	1 oz._____	28	8	115	1	4
534	Gum drops_____	1 oz._____	28	12	100	Trace	Trace
535	Hard_____	1 oz._____	28	1	110	0	Trace
536	Marshmallows_____	1 oz._____	28	17	90	1	Trace

EDIBLE PART OF FOODS *(continued)*

	Fatty acids		Carbo-hydrate	Cal-cium	Iron	Vita-min A value	Thia-min	Ribo-flavin	Niacin	Ascor-bic acid
Satu-rated (total)	Unsaturated									
	Oleic	Lin-oleic								
Grams	Grams	Grams	Grams	Milli-grams	Milli-grams	Inter-national units	Milli-grams	Milli-grams	Milli-grams	Milli-grams
1	1	3	3	2	.1					
-------	-------	-------	Trace	2	.1					
1	1	Trace	2	14	.1	80	.01	.03	Trace	Trace
2	2	6	Trace	3	.1	40	Trace	.01	Trace	------
1	2	4	3	2	.1	50	Trace	Trace	Trace	Trace
21	14	1	185	165	3.3	580	.06	.28	.6	1
11	1	Trace	124	10	.8	0	.02	.07	.3	0
5	8	3	183	96	2.7	Trace	.05	.20	.7	Trace
-------	-------	-------	76	2	Trace	0	Trace	.03	Trace	0
2	1	Trace	22	42	.4	Trace	.01	.05	.1	Trace
5	3	Trace	16	65	.3	80	.02	.10	.1	Trace
3	6	2	11	33	.4	Trace	.10	.05	2.1	Trace
-------	-------	-------	25	4	.3	0	Trace	Trace	Trace	0
2	1	Trace	21	22	.3	Trace	.01	.03	.1	Trace
			25	2	.1	0	0	Trace	Trace	0
			28	6	.5	0	0	0	0	0
			23	5	.5	0	0	Trace	Trace	0

TABLE 1.—NUTRITIVE VALUES OF THE

Food, approximate measure, and weight (in grams)			Water	Food energy	Pro-tein	Fat
VEGETABLES AND VEGETABLE PRODUCTS—Continued						
SUGARS, SWEETS		Grams	Per-cent	Calo-ries	Grams	Grams
	Chocolate-flavored sirup or topping:					
537	Thin type	1 fl. oz. 38	32	90	1	1
538	Fudge type	1 fl. oz. 38	25	125	2	5
	Chocolate-flavored beverage powder (approx. 4 heaping teaspoons per oz.):					
539	With nonfat dry milk	1 oz. 28	2	100	5	1
540	Without nonfat dry milk.	1 oz. 28	1	100	1	1
541	Honey, strained or extracted.	1 tbsp. 21	17	65	Trace	0
542	Jams and preserves	1 tbsp. 20	29	55	Trace	Trace
543	Jellies	1 tbsp. 18	29	50	Trace	Trace
	Molasses, cane:					
544	Light (first extraction)	1 tbsp. 20	24	50	------	------
545	Blackstrap (third extraction).	1 tbsp. 20	24	45	------	------
	Sirups:					
546	Sorghum	1 tbsp. 21	23	55	------	------
547	Table blends, chiefly corn, light and dark.	1 tbsp. 21	24	60	0	0
	Sugars:					
548	Brown, firm packed	1 cup 220	2	820	0	0
	White:					
549	Granulated	1 cup 200	Trace	770	0	0
550		1 tbsp. 11	Trace	40	0	0
551	Powdered, stirred before measuring.	1 cup 120	Trace	460	0	0

Fatty acids			Carbo-hy-drate	Cal-cium	Iron	Vita-min A value	Thia-min	Ribo-flavin	Niacin	Ascor-bic acid
Satu-rated (total)	Unsaturated									
	Oleic	Lin-oleic								
Grams	*Grams*	*Grams*	*Grams*	*Milli-grams*	*Milli-grams*	*Inter-national units*	*Milli-grams*	*Milli-grams*	*Milli-grams*	*Milli-grams*
Trace	Trace	Trace	24	6	.6	Trace	.01	.03	.2	0
3	2	Trace	20	48	.5	60	.02	.08	.2	Trace
Trace	Trace	Trace	20	167	.5	10	.04	.21	.2	1
Trace	Trace	Trace	25	9	.6	-------	.01	.03	.1	0
------	------	------	17	1	.1	0	Trace	.01	.1	Trace
------	------	------	14	4	.2	Trace	Trace	.01	Trace	Trace
------	------	------	13	4	.3	Trace	Trace	.01	Trace	1
------	------	------	13	33	.9	-------	.01	.01	Trace	------
------	------	------	11	137	3.2	-------	.02	.04	.4	------
------	------	------	14	35	2.6	-------	-------	.02	Trace	------
------	------	------	15	9	.8	0	0	0	0	0
------	------	------	212	187	7.5	0	.02	.07	.4	0
------	------	------	199	0	.2	0	0	0	0	0
------	------	------	11	0	Trace	0	0	0	0	0
------	------	------	119	0	.1	0	0	0	0	0

TABLE 1.—NUTRITIVE VALUES OF THE

	Food, approximate measure, and weight (in grams)		Water	Food energy	Protein	Fat
	MISCELLANEOUS ITEMS	*Grams*	*Percent*	*Calories*	*Grams*	*Grams*
552	Barbecue sauce_____ 1 cup_____	250	81	230	4	17
	Beverages, alcoholic:					
553	Beer_____ 12 fl. oz._____	360	92	150	1	0
	Gin, rum, vodka, whiskey:					
554	80-proof_____ 1½ fl. oz. jigger.	42	67	100	_____	_____
555	86-proof_____ 1½ fl. oz. jigger.	42	64	105	_____	_____
556	90-proof_____ 1½ fl. oz. jigger.	42	62	110	_____	_____
557	94-proof_____ 1½ fl. oz. jigger.	42	60	115	_____	_____
558	100-proof_____ 1½ fl. oz. jigger.	42	58	125	_____	_____
	Wines:					
559	Dessert_____ 3½ fl. oz. glass.	103	77	140	Trace	0
560	Table_____ 3½ fl. oz. glass.	102	86	85	Trace	0
	Beverages, carbonated, sweetened, nonalcoholic:					
561	Carbonated water_____ 12 fl. oz._____	366	92	115	0	0
562	Cola type_____ 12 fl. oz._____	369	90	145	0	0
563	Fruit-flavored sodas and Tom Collins mixes. 12 fl. oz._____	372	88	170	0	0
564	Ginger ale_____ 12 fl. oz._____	366	92	115	0	0
565	Root beer_____ 12 fl. oz._____	370	90	150	0	0
566	Bouillon cubes, approx. 1 cube_____ ½ in.	4	4	5	1	Trace

EDIBLE PART OF FOODS *(continued)*

	Fatty acids		Carbo-hy-drate	Cal-cium	Iron	Vita-min A value	Thia-min	Ribo-flavin	Niacin	Ascor-bic acid
Satu-rated (total)	Unsaturated									
	Oleic	Lin-oleic								
Grams	*Grams*	*Grams*	*Grams*	*Milli-grams*	*Milli-grams*	*Inter-national units*	*Milli-grams*	*Milli-grams*	*Milli-grams*	*Milli-grams*
2	5	9	20	53	2.0	900	.03	.03	.8	13
------	------	------	14	18	Trace	-------	.01	.11	2.2	------
------	------	------	Trace	------	------	------	------	------	------	------
------	------	------	Trace	------	------	------	------	------	------	------
------	------	------	Trace	------	------	------	------	------	------	------
------	------	------	Trace	------	------	------	------	------	------	------
------	------	------	Trace	------	------	------	------	------	------	------
------	------	------	8	8	------	------	.01	.02	.2	------
------	------	------	4	9	.4	------	Trace	.01	.1	------
------	------	------	29	------	------	0	0	0	0	0
------	------	------	37	------	------	0	0	0	0	0
------	------	------	45	------	------	0	0	0	0	0
------	------	------	29	------	------	0	0	0	0	0
------	------	------	39	------	------	0	0	0	0	0
------	------	------	Trace	------	------	------	------	------	------	------

TABLE 1.—NUTRITIVE VALUES OF THE

	Food, approximate measure, and weight (in grams)		Water	Food energy	Pro-tein	Fat
		Grams	Per-cent	Calo-ries	Grams	Grams

MISCELLANEOUS ITEMS—Continued

			Grams	Per-cent	Calo-ries	Grams	Grams
	Chocolate:						
567	Bitter or baking	1 oz.	28	2	145	3	15
568	Semi-sweet, small pieces.	1 cup	170	1	860	7	61
	Gelatin:						
569	Plain, dry powder in envelope.	1 envelope	7	13	25	6	Trace
570	Dessert powder, 3-oz. package.	1 pkg.	85	2	315	8	0
571	Gelatin dessert, prepared with water.	1 cup	240	84	140	4	0
	Olives, pickled:						
572	Green	4 medium or 3 extra large or 2 giant.	16	78	15	Trace	2
573	Ripe: Mission	3 small or 2 large.	10	73	15	Trace	2
	Pickles, cucumber:						
574	Dill, medium, whole, 3¾ in. long, 1¼ in. diam.	1 pickle	65	93	10	1	Trace
575	Fresh, sliced, 1½ in. diam., ¼ in. thick.	2 slices	15	79	10	Trace	Trace
576	Sweet, gherkin, small, whole, approx. 2½ in. long, ¾ in. diam.	1 pickle	15	61	20	Trace	Trace
577	Relish, finely chopped, sweet.	1 tbsp.	15	63	20	Trace	Trace
	Popcorn. See Grain Products.						
578	Popsicle, 3 fl. oz. size	1 popsicle	95	80	70	0	0

EDIBLE PART OF FOODS *(continued)*

Fatty acids			Carbo-hy-drate	Cal-cium	Iron	Vita-min A value	Thia-min	Ribo-flavin	Niacin	Ascor-bic acid
Satu-rated (total)	Unsaturated									
	Oleic	Lin-oleic								
Grams	*Grams*	*Grams*	*Grams*	*Milli-grams*	*Milli-grams*	*Inter-national units*	*Milli-grams*	*Milli-grams*	*Milli-grams*	*Milli-grams*
8	6	Trace	8	22	1.9	20	.01	.07	.4	0
34	22	1	97	51	4.4	30	.02	.14	.9	0
------	------	------	0	------	------	------	------	------	------	------
------	------	------	75	------	------	------	------	------	------	------
------	------	------	34	------	------	------	------	------	------	------
Trace	2	Trace	Trace	8	.2	40	------	------	------	------
Trace	2	Trace	Trace	9	.1	10	Trace	Trace	------	------
------	------	------	1	17	.7	70	Trace	.01	Trace	4
------	------	------	3	5	.3	20	Trace	Trace	Trace	1
------	------	------	6	2	.2	10	Trace	Trace	Trace	1
------	------	------	5	3	.1	------	------	------	------	------
0	0	0	18	0	Trace	0	0	0	0	0

TABLE 1.—NUTRITIVE VALUES OF THE

	Food, approximate measure, and weight (in grams)			Water	Food energy	Pro- tein	Fat

			Grams	Per- cent	Calo- ries	Grams	Grams
	Pudding, home recipe with starch base:						
579	Chocolate............	1 cup........	260	66	385	8	12
580	Vanilla (blanc mange)..	1 cup........	255	76	285	9	10
581	Pudding mix, dry form, 4-oz. package.	1 pkg........	113	2	410	3	2
582	Sherbet.................	1 cup........	193	67	260	2	2
	Soups:						
	Canned, condensed, ready-to-serve:						
	Prepared with an equal volume of milk:						
583	Cream of chicken..	1 cup........	245	85	180	7	10
584	Cream of mush- room.	1 cup........	245	83	215	7	14
585	Tomato..........	1 cup........	250	84	175	7	7
	Prepared with an equal volume of water:						
586	Bean with pork....	1 cup........	250	84	170	8	6
587	Beef broth, bouil- lon consomme.	1 cup........	240	96	30	5	0
588	Beef noodle........	1 cup........	240	93	70	4	3
589	Clam chowder, Manhattan type (with tomatoes, without milk).	1 cup........	245	92	80	2	3
590	Cream of chicken..	1 cup........	240	92	95	3	6
591	Cream of mush- room.	1 cup........	240	90	135	2	10
592	Minestrone........	1 cup........	245	90	105	5	3
593	Split pea..........	1 cup........	245	85	145	9	3
594	Tomato...........	1 cup........	245	90	90	2	3
595	Vegetable beef....	1 cup........	245	92	80	5	2
596	Vegetarian........	1 cup........	245	92	80	2	2

EDIBLE PART OF FOODS (continued)

Fatty acids			Carbo-hy-drate	Cal-cium	Iron	Vita-min A value	Thia-min	Ribo-flavin	Niacin	Ascor-bic acid
Satu-rated (total)	Unsaturated									
	Oleic	Lin-oleic								
Grams	Grams	Grams	Grams	Milli-grams	Milli-grams	Inter-national units	Milli-grams	Milli-grams	Milli-grams	Milli-grams
7	4	Trace	67	250	1.3	390	.05	.36	.3	1
5	3	Trace	41	298	Trace	410	.08	.41	.3	2
1	1	Trace	103	23	1.8	Trace	.02	.08	.5	0
------	------	------	59	31	Trace	120	.02	.06	Trace	4
3	3	3	15	172	.5	610	.05	.27	.7	2
4	4	5	16	191	.5	250	.05	.34	.7	1
3	2	1	23	168	.8	1,200	.10	.25	1.3	15
1	2	2	22	63	2.3	650	.13	.08	1.0	3
			3	Trace	.5	Trace	Trace	.02	1.2	------
1	1	1	7	7	1.0	50	.05	.07	1.0	Trace
------	------	------	12	34	1.0	880	.02	.02	1.0	------
1	2	3	8	24	.5	410	.02	.05	.5	Trace
1	3	5	10	41	.5	70	.02	.12	.7	Trace
------	------	------	14	37	1.0	2,350	.07	.05	1.0	------
1	2	Trace	21	29	1.5	440	0.25	0.15	1.5	1
Trace	1	1	16	15	.7	1,000	.05	.05	1.2	12
------	------	------	10	12	.7	2,700	.05	.05	1.0	------
------	------	------	13	20	1.0	2,940	.05	.05	1.0	------

TABLE 1.—NUTRITIVE VALUES OF THE

	Food, approximate measure, and weight (in grams)			Water	Food energy	Pro-tein	Fat
	MISCELLANEOUS ITEMS—Continued						
	Soups—Continued		Grams	Per-cent	Calo-ries	Grams	Grams
	Dehydrated, dry form:						
597	Chicken noodle (2-oz. package).	1 pkg.	57	6	220	8	6
598	Onion mix (1½-oz. package).	1 pkg.	43	3	150	6	5
599	Tomato vegetable with noodles (2½-oz. pkg.).	1 pkg.	71	4	245	6	6
	Frozen, condensed:						
	Clam chowder, New England type (with milk, without tomatoes):						
600	Prepared with equal volume of milk.	1 cup	245	83	210	9	12
601	Prepared with equal volume of water.	1 cup	240	89	130	4	8
	Cream of potato:						
602	Prepared with equal volume of milk.	1 cup	245	83	185	8	10
603	Prepared with equal volume of water.	1 cup	240	90	105	3	5
	Cream of shrimp:						
604	Prepared with equal volume of milk.	1 cup	245	82	245	9	16
605	Prepared with equal volume of water.	1 cup	240	88	160	5	12

EDIBLE PART OF FOODS (continued)

Fatty acids			Carbo-hy-drate	Cal-cium	Iron	Vita-min A value	Thia-min	Ribo-flavin	Niacin	Ascor-bic acid
Satu-rated (total)	Unsaturated									
	Oleic	Lin-oleic								
Grams	Grams	Grams	Grams	Milli-grams	Milli-grams	Inter-national units	Milli-grams	Milli-grams	Milli-grams	Milli-grams
2	3	1	33	34	1.4	190	.30	.15	2.4	3
1	2	1	23	42	.6	30	.05	.03	.3	6
2	3	1	45	33	1.4	1,700	.21	.13	1.8	18
------	------	------	16	240	1.0	250	.07	.29	.5	Trace
------	------	------	11	91	1.0	50	.05	.10	.5	------
5	3	Trace	18	208	1.0	590	.10	.27	.5	Trace
3	2	Trace	12	58	1.0	410	.05	.05	.5	------
------	------	------	15	189	.5	290	.07	.27	.5	Trace
------	------	------	8	38	.5	120	.05	.05	.5	------

TABLE 1.—NUTRITIVE VALUES OF THE

Food, approximate measure, and weight (in grams)			Water	Food energy	Pro-tein	Fat
MISCELLANEOUS ITEMS—Continued						
Soups—Continued		*Grams*	*Per-cent*	*Calo-ries*	*Grams*	*Grams*
	Oyster stew:					
606	Prepared with equal volume of milk.	1 cup_____ 240	83	200	10	12
607	Prepared with equal volume of water.	1 cup_____ 240	90	120	6	8
608	Tapioca, dry, quick-cooking.	1 cup_____ 152	13	535	1	Trace
	Tapioca desserts:					
609	Apple_____ 1 cup_____	250	70	295	1	Trace
610	Cream pudding_____ 1 cup_____	165	72	220	8	8
611	Tartar sauce_____ 1 tbsp_____	14	34	75	Trace	8
612	Vinegar_____ 1 tbsp_____	15	94	Trace	Trace	0
613	White sauce, medium____ 1 cup_____	250	73	405	10	31
	Yeast:					
614	Baker's, dry, active____ 1 pkg_____	7	5	20	3	Trace
615	Brewer's, dry_____ 1 tbsp_____	8	5	25	3	Trace
	Yoghurt. See Milk, Cheese, Cream, Imitation Cream.					

EDIBLE PART OF FOODS *(continued)*

Fatty acids			Carbo-hydrate	Cal-cium	Iron	Vita-min A value	Thia-min	Ribo-flavin	Niacin	Ascor-bic acid
Satu-rated (total)	Unsaturated									
	Oleic	Lin-oleic								
Grams	*Grams*	*Grams*	*Grams*	*Milli-grams*	*Milli-grams*	*Inter-national units*	*Milli-grams*	*Milli-grams*	*Milli-grams*	*Milli-grams*
------	------	------	14	305	1.4	410	.12	.41	.5	Trace
------	------	------	8	158	1.4	240	.07	.19	.5	------
------	------	------	131	15	.6	0	0	0	0	0
------	------	------	74	8	.5	30	Trace	Trace	Trace	Trace
4	3	Trace	28	173	.7	480	.07	.30	.2	2
1	1	4	1	3	.1	30	Trace	Trace	Trace	Trace
------	------	------	1	1	.1	------	------	------	------	------
16	10	1	22	288	.5	1,150	.10	.43	.5	2
------	------	------	3	3	1.1	Trace	.16	.38	2.6	Trace
------	------	------	3	17	1.4	Trace	1.25	.34	3.0	Trace

YIELD OF COOKED MEAT

Meat as purchased

Chops or steaks for broiling or frying:
With bone and relatively large amount of fat, such as pork or lamb chops; beef rib, sirloin, or porterhouse steaks.

Without bone and with very little fat, such as round of beef, veal steaks_____

Ground meat for broiling or frying, such as beef, lamb, or pork patties_____

Roasts for oven cooking (no liquid added):
With bone and relatively large amount of fat, such as beef rib, loin, chuck; lamb shoulder, leg; pork, fresh or cured.

Without bone_____

Cuts for pot-roasting, simmering, braising, stewing:
With bone and relatively large amount of fat, such as beef chuck, pork shoulder_

Without bone and with relatively small amount of fat, such as trimmed beef, veal.

PER POUND OF RAW MEAT

Meat after cooking (less drippings)	
Parts weighed	Approximate weight of cooked parts per pound of raw meat purchased
	Ounces
Lean, bone, fat_____	10–12
Lean and fat_____	7–10
Lean only_____	5–7
Lean and fat_____	12–13
Lean only_____	9–12
Patties_____	9–13
Lean, bone, fat_____	10–12
Lean and fat_____	8–10
Lean only_____	6–9
Lean and fat_____	10–12
Lean only_____	7–10
Lean, bone, fat_____	10–11
Lean and fat_____	8–9
Lean only_____	6–8
Lean with adhering fat_____	9–11

TABLE 2.—RECOMMENDED DAILY DIETARY ALLOWANCES (*abridged*)[1]

(Designed for the maintenance of good nutrition of practically all healthy persons in the U.S.A.)

	Age (years)	Weight (kg)	Weight (lbs)	Height (cm)	Height (in)	Energy (kcal)	Protein (g)	Vitamin A (IU)	Ascorbic Acid (mg)	Niacin (mg)	Riboflavin (mg)	Thiamin (mg)	Calcium (grams)	Iron (mg)
Infants	0.0–0.5	6	14	60	24	kg × 117	kg × 2.2	1,400	35	5	0.4	0.3	360	10
	0.5–1.0	9	20	71	28	kg × 108	kg × 2.0	2,000	35	8	0.6	0.5	540	15
Children	1–3	13	28	86	34	1,300	23	2,000	40	9	0.8	0.7	800	15
	4–6	20	44	110	44	1,800	30	2,500	40	12	1.1	0.9	800	10
	7–10	30	66	135	54	2,400	36	3,300	40	16	1.2	1.2	800	10
Males	11–14	44	97	158	63	2,800	44	5,000	45	18	1.5	1.4	1,200	18
	15–18	61	134	172	69	3,000	54	5,000	45	20	1.8	1.5	1,200	18
	19–22	67	147	172	69	3,000	54	5,000	45	20	1.8	1.5	800	10
	23–50	70	154	172	69	2,700	56	5,000	45	18	1.6	1.4	800	10
	51+	70	154	172	69	2,400	56	5,000	45	16	1.5	1.2	800	10
Females	11–14	44	97	155	62	2,400	44	4,000	45	16	1.3	1.2	1,200	18
	15–18	54	119	162	65	2,100	48	4,000	45	14	1.4	1.1	1,200	18
	19–22	58	128	162	65	2,100	46	4,000	45	14	1.4	1.1	800	18
	23–50	58	128	162	65	2,000	46	4,000	45	13	1.2	1.0	800	18
	51+	58	128	162	65	1,800	46	4,000	45	12	1.1	1.0	800	10
Pregnant						+300	+30	5,000	60	+2	+0.3	+0.3	1,200	18+
Lactating						+500	+20	6,000	80	+4	+0.5	+0.3	1,200	18

FOR FURTHER READING

NUTRITION

Nutrition And Physical Fitness, by L. Jean Bogert, Ph.D., and others, W. B. Saunders Company, 1973.
  —a textbook on nutrients and health.
Nutrition, by Margaret S. Chaney and Margaret L. Ross, Houghton Mifflin Company, 1971.
  —another textbook, with greater emphasis on chemistry.
Recommended Dietary Allowances, The National Academy of Sciences, 1974.
  —the standards for the nutrients and how they are set.
Nutritive Value of American Foods, Agriculture Handbook No. 456, The United States Department of Agriculture, 1975.
  —the foods we eat and their nutritive values in common servings.

ENERGY AND OVERWEIGHT

Overweight, by Jean Mayer, Prentice-Hall, Inc., 1968.
  —the definitive text on obesity and all its aspects.

Energetics, by Grant Gwinup, M.D., Bantam Books, 1970.
    —an easy-to-read popular discussion of the relationship
        between food energy, physical activity, and the control
        of fat on the human body.

DIETING

Rating The Diets, by Theodore Berland and the Editors of Consumer Guide, Consumer Guide, 1977.
    —a guide to the popular diet plans and their worth to the
        dieter; the author, however, is a little confused over
        low-carbohydrate diets and their value to weight
        reduction—otherwise, very good.

EXERCISE

Aerobics, by Kenneth H. Cooper, M.D., Bantam Books, 1968.
    —Dr. Cooper describes how to exercise for maximal
        health and fitness benefits.
The New Aerobics, by Kenneth H. Cooper, M.D., Bantam Books, 1970.
    —Dr. Cooper updates his excellent earlier work.
Aerobics for Women, by Mildred Cooper and Kenneth H. Cooper, M.D., Bantam Books, 1972.
    —exercise programs with the ladies in mind.

A NOTE FROM THE AUTHOR

Can I make the claim that *Diet With Vitamins* is the last word on weight reduction?

Well, science has a way of advancing.

The perimeters of our knowledge always seem to expand.

Yet, as of this moment, and undoubtedly for many years to come, the information and methods of reducing presented here will remain valid and the best available, for the principles and physical laws that form the basis of the natural vitamin way will not change. In this respect, they're like Einstein's law of energy and matter—not to be denied. Certainly research will make small breakthroughs here and solve another mystery there, always adding bits and pieces; but the foundations will remain the same, and thus the system will forever work.

With this in mind, then, you can rely on the information and instructions in *Diet With Vitamins*, confident that for now and the foreseeable future, on how to lose weight and improve your health and looks, it is the last word.

INDEX

Aging and Vitamin E, 67
Alcoholism, 55
Amino acids, 59, 83, 84, 85, 168
Amphetamines, 101
Anemia
    biotin deficiency and, 76
    copper and, 77
    folacin deficiency and, 27, 72
    indications of, 44
    iron deficiency and, 44
    macroytic, 72
    pernicious, 75
    prevention of, 77
    vitamin B-6 deficiency and, 74
    vitamin E deficiency and, 68
Antacids, 77
Appestat, 93–94, 97, 156
Arteriosclerosis, 82
Ascorbic acid, 33, 37
Atkins, Dr. Robert, 104
Atrophy, 84
Avidin, 76
Avitaminosis, 25

Baking soda, 40, 57
Basal metabolic rate, 91, 100
Beriberi, 18, 53–54, 55, 56
Bile fluids, 82

Bioflavinoids, 17
Biotin, 16, 75–76
Blindness, 24, 25, 63
Blood clotting
    calcium and, 49
    vitamin K deficiency and, 73
Bones
    calcium and, 18, 49
    damage to, 26
    phosphorus and, 76, 77
Bortz, Walter, 105
Boussingault, 42
Brain
    appestat and, 93
    cholesterol and, 82–83
    hunger and, 93
    hypothalamus and, 93
Brown rice and tea diet, 20

Calcium, 48–52
    blood clotting and, 49
    bones and, 18, 49
    deficiency of, 50–51
    diet plans and, 51
    discovery of, 48
    functions of, 49
    milk and, 52, 141
    minerals and, 18

Calcium (*cont.*)
  phosphate, 48
  phosphorus and, 77
  RDA, 51
  sources of, 52
  sulfate, 48
  teeth and, 48, 50
  vegetables and, 52
  vitamin B-12 and, 51
Calorie(s)
  basal metabolic rate and, 91
  carbohydrates vs., 104
  daily expenditure tables, 118–129
  deficit, 99
  demand for, 102
  dieting and, 91
  energy and, 91
  exercise and, 92, 99, 155
  fat and, 81, 91
  output, 112
  overweight and, 89
  sources of, 15
  study on, 105
Carbohydrates, 79–81
  calories vs., 104
  cellulose, 79
  composition of, 79
  diet, 80, 104
  energy nutrients, 78
  glucose and, 79
  glycogen and, 80
  necessity of, 79, 81
  sodium retention and, 107
  sources of, 81
  thiamin and, 55
Carotene, 22–23, 59
Cartilage, 33
Cellulose, 79, 80
Chlorine, 76
Cholesterol
  arteriosclerosis and, 82
  bile fluids and, 82
  brain composition and, 82–83
  nicotinic acid and, 60
  vitamin D transformation and, 71, 82
Choline, 16, 73–74
Chossat, 48
Coagulation, 73
Colds and Vitamin C, 35–36
Collagen (protein), 33

Coronary disease, 60
Cretinism, 70
Cryptoxanthin, 22–23

Davy, Sir Humphry, 48
Decalcification, 50
Diabetes, 60, 157
Diarrhea
  fat overbundance and, 83
  niacin deficiency and, 26
  pellagra and, 11
  vitamin C and, 37
Deficiency of
  biotin, 76
  calcium, 50–51
  fiber, 80, 81
  folacin, 27
  hemoglobin, 44
  iodine, 70
  iron, 41, 43–45, 69–70
  niacin, 16, 18, 26, 60
  pantothenic acid, 75
  phosphorus, 77
  protein, 25, 84
  riboflavin, 63–64
  thiamin, 54
  vitamin A, 24–25, 26
  vitamin B-6, 74
  vitamin B-12, 75
  vitamin C, 18, 29–30, 34–35
  vitamin D, 71
  vitamin E, 67, 68
  vitamin K, 73
Dieting
  amino acids, necessity in, 85
  amphetamines and, 101
  calories and, 99
  defective, 15
  drugs and, 100
  injections and, 100
  iodine and, 70
  iron deficiency and, 44–45
  machines and, 102
  niacin and, 60
  nutrients and, 10
  pills and, 101
  polyunsaturated fat and, 82
  protein, necessity in 84–85
  RDA and, 20–21, 28

Dieting (*cont.*)
  schemes, 1–2
  science and, 3, 89, 108
  surgery and, 102
  weight control clinics, 100
Diet plans, 111–149
  calcium and, 51
  food baskets, 145–149
  grapefruit, 101
  how to use, 115–117, 142–143
  low-carbohydrate, 80, 104
  menus, 130–139, 145–149
  nutritional data on, 151–154
  science and, 6
Dissacharides, 79
Diuretic, 101
Diverticula, 81
Diverticulitis, 81

Eijkman, Christian, 53–54
Energy and the human body, 90–91
Energy nutrients. *See* carbohydrates, fat
  and protein.
Exercise
  appestat and, 94, 156
  beginning, 157–159
  calories and, 92, 99, 155
  effect of, 156
  jogging, 161
  running in place, 160–161
  schemes, 1–2
  technology and, 95–97
  tips on, 160–162
  walking, 155, 157, 160
  weight reduction and, 155–162

Fasting, 140
Fat, 81–82
Fat-soluble vitamins, 16
Fiber, 79, 80, 81
Folacin,
  deficiency of, 27
  nucleic acid synthesis and, 72
  RDA, 73
  sources of, 73, 168
  water-soluble vitamin, 16
Food
  measure of, 164

Food (*cont.*)
  values, 165
  value table, 163, 254
Food and Drug Administration, 19
Food-faddists, 16–17, 55–56
Food and Nutrition Board of National
  Academy of Sciences, 19, 45, 73
Fructose, 79
Fruits and Vitamin C, 31–32
Funk, Casimir, 15

Galactose, 79
Glucose, 79
Glycogen, 80
Goiters and iodine deficiency, 69–70
Goldberger, Joseph, 12–14, 58
Grapefruit diet, 101

HCG, 100
Hemoglobin, 18, 42, 44
Hemorrhoids, 43
High blood pressure and salt, 76
High protein diets, 103
Holmes, William L., 105
Howat, Paula, 105
Huber, 58
Hypothalamus, 93
Hypervitaminosis A, 26
Hypovitaminosis A, 25

Infection and Vitamin C, 34
Insulin, 83
Intestines, removal of, 103
Iodine
  basal metabolic rate, 69
  cretinism, 70
  deficiency, 70
  dieting and, 70
  iodized salt, 70
  overdosage, 70
  sources of, 168
  thyroid hormones and, 69
Iron
  anemia, 44
  deficiency, 41, 43–45
  hemoglobin and, 18, 42, 44
  oxygen and, 42–43

Iron (*cont.*)
  pills, 46
  poisoning, 46
  RDA, 45, 46, 141
  source of, 141
  storage of, 42, 43

Jogging, 161

Ketones, 80
Ketosis, 80
Korsakoff's Disease, 55
Kwashiorkor (protein deficiency), 25

Lactose, 79
Latent scurvy, 34
Lind, James, 15, 31
Linear programming, 141
Linoleic acid, 82
Liver, 23
Low-carbohydrate diet, 80, 104, 107

Macrocytic anemia, 72
Magnesium, 77, 168
Mal de la rosa, 10
Mayer, Jean, 161
MDR (Minimum Daily Requirements), 19
Menus, 130–139, 145–149
Mexican typhus fever, 12
Milk,
  calcium source, 52, 141
  iron source, 141
  lactose, 79
  protein, 141
  tryptophan in, 59
Minerals
  calcium, 18
  chlorine, 76
  defined, 18
  iron, 41–47
  magnesium, 77
  necessity in diet, 3, 15
  phosphorus, 77
  potassium, 77
  sodium, 76

Mucous membranes, 24
Multiple sclerosis, 64, 66

Niacin
  alcoholics and, 60
  beriberi and, 59
  coronary disease and, 60
  deficiency, 16, 18, 26, 60
  dieting and, 60
  discovery of, 14
  overdoses of, 26, 60
  pellagra and, 14, 16, 18, 58, 60
  RDA, 60
  sources of, 61
  table, 254
  tuberculosis and, 60
  values, 168, 254
  water-soluble vitamin, 16, 26, 61
Nicotinamide, 58
Nicotinic acid, 58, 60
Nightblindness, 24
Nitrogen, 84, 85, 140
Nucleic acid synthesis, 72
Nutrient, 9
  classes of, 78
  defined, 78
  dieting and, 10
  discovery of, 15
  energy, 78
  niacin, 14

Obesity, 89–98
Osteoporosis, 50–51
Oxidation, 23, 40, 68

Pantothenic acid, 16, 75
Pasteur, Louis, 13
Pauling, Linus, 35
Pellagra, 11–14, 16, 18, 58, 60
Pernicious anemia, 75
Phosphorus, 77, 168
Physical fitness and exercise, 157–162
Placebo, 37
Polyunsaturated fat, 82, 83
Potassium, 77
Potato, 39

Protein
  amino acids, 83
  avidin, 76
  collagen, 33
  deficiency, 25, 84
  diet, 103
  duties of, 83
  energy nutrient, 78
  milk and, 141
  necessity of, 84–85
  nitrogen and, 84, 85, 140
  overdosage, 85
  RDA, 84, 85, 140
Publications on nutrients, 169
Pyruvic acid, 55

RDA (Recommended Dietary Allowances)
  biotin, 76
  calcium, 51
  carbohydrates, 81
  choline, 74
  daily requirements, 19
  diet plans and, 116, 142
  dieting and, 20–21, 28
  fiber, 81
  folacin, 73
  iodine, 70
  iron, 43, 45, 46, 141
  meeting requirements of, 116
  niacin, 60
  pantothenic acid, 75
  protein, 84, 85, 140
  riboflavin, 64
  thiamin, 56
  tryptophan, 60
  vitamin A, 27
  vitamin B-6, 74
  vitamin B-12, 75
  vitamin C, 35, 38, 39
  vitamin D, 72
  vitamin E, 67
  vitamin K, 73
Recommended Daily Dietary
    Allowances, 167, 255
Red sickness, 10
Reproduction, 24, 66, 76
Retinol, 23
Riboflavin, 16, 63–64
Rickets, 71

Saturated fat, 82
Scurvy, 15, 29–32, 34
SDA (Specific Dynamic Action), 103
Skin disorders and Vitamin E, 66
Sodium
  carbohydrates and, 107
  chlorine and, 76
  depletion, 76
  diets and, 107
  high blood pressure and, 76
  necessity of, 76
Sources of
  biotin, 75
  calcium, 52
  calories, 15
  carbohydrates, 81
  choline, 74
  folacin, 73, 168
  iodine, 70, 168
  iron, 141
  niacin, 61
  pantothenic acid, 75
  phosphorus, 168
  polyunsaturated fat, 83
  thiamin, 56–57
  vitamin A, 23
  vitamin B-6, 74, 167
  vitamin B-12, 74, 168
  vitamin C, 38–39
  vitamin D, 71, 168
  vitamin E, 68, 168
  vitamin K, 73
Starch, 79
Stillman Diet, 103–104
Stillman, Irwin, 103
Sucrose, 79
Sugars, 79

Teeth
  calcium and, 48, 50
  phosphorus and, 76
  vitamin C and, 29–31
  vitamin D and, 71
Thiamin
  alcoholics and, 55
  beriberi and, 18, 53–54, 55
  carbohydrates and, 55
  deficiency, 54
  destruction of, 57

Thiamin (*cont.*)
  discovery of, 15
  food-faddists and, 55–56
  functions of, 54–55
  Korsakoff's disease, 55
  pills, 26
  RDA, 56
  sources of, 56–57
  storage of, 56
  synthetic, 56
  water-soluble vitamin, 16, 56
  Wernicke's disease, 55
  yeast, 57
Thyroid hormones, 69, 70
Tryptophan, 59, 60, 63, 84, 168
Tuberculosis, 60

USDA (United States Department of
    Agriculture), 169

Vegetables
  As sources of:
    calcium, 52
    folacin, 73
    value of, 165
    vitamin A, 23
    vitamin C, 38–40
    vitamin E, 68
    vitamin K, 73
Vision and
  riboflavin, 63
  vitamin A, 23–24
  Wernicke's disease, 55
Vitamin
  defined, 16
  deficiency of, 26
  discovery of, 26
  MDR, 19
  necessity of, 3–4
  overdose of, 26
  origin of name, 15
  pills, 25–27, 34–35
  RDA, 19
  role of, 16–18
Vitamin A, 22–28
  bones and teeth and, 24
  deficiency, 24–26
  destruction of, 23
  discovery of, 22

Vitamin A (*cont.*)
  fat-soluble, 16, 23, 26
  malnutrition and, 25
  mucous membranes and, 24
  overdosage, 26
  oxidation, 23, 66
  pills, 25–26
  RDA, 27
  reproduction and, 24
  retinol and, 23
  role of, 23–25
  sources of, 23
  storage, 23, 26
  vision and, 23–25
Vitamin B–2 *See* Riboflavin.
Vitamin B-6
  deficiency, 74
  RDA, 74
  source of, 74, 167
  water-soluble, 16, 74
Vitamin B-12
  calcium and, 51
  deficiency, 75
  RDA, 75
  sources, 74, 168
  water-soluble, 16, 74
Vitamin C, 29–40
  cartilage and, 33
  characteristics, 33
  colds and, 35–36
  collagen and, 33
  deficiency, 18, 29–30, 34–35
  destruction of, 40
  fruits and, 31–32
  healing of wounds and, 33
  importance of, 33–34
  latent scurvy, 34
  overdose, 34, 38
  RDA, 35, 38, 39
  scurvy, 29–32
  sources of, 38–39
  teeth and, 29–31
  water-soluble, 16
Vitamin D
  cholesterol and, 82
  deficiency of, 71
  discovery of, 71
  fat-soluble, 16, 71
  overdose, 71
  RDA, 71
  rickets and, 71

Vitamin D (*cont.*)
  source of, 71, 168
  teeth and, 71
Vitamin E
  aging and, 67
  antitoxidant, 66
  athletic ability and, 67
  characteristics, 66
  deficiency, 67
  dieting and, 67–68
  fat-soluble, 16, 66
  multiple sclerosis and, 64, 66
  overdose, 67
  preservative, 68
  reproduction and, 66
  RDA, 67
  skin disorders and, 66
  sources, 68, 168
Vitamin G. *See* Riboflavin.

Vitamin K
  blood clotting and, 73
  deficiency, 73
  fat-soluble, 16, 73
  RDA, 73
  source of, 73

Water-soluble vitamins, 16
Wernicke's disease, 55

xerophthalmia, 24

Yeast, 57

Zen Macrobiotic Plan, 4, 20